# 1001

## Ways to

## Anxiety
## Relief

# 1001

## Ways to

# Anxiety Relief

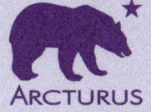

ARCTURUS

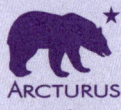

ARCTURUS

This edition published in 2025 by Arcturus Publishing Limited
26/27 Bickels Yard, 151–153 Bermondsey Street,
London SE1 3HA

ISBN: 978-1-3988-6025-4
AD012874NT

Printed in China

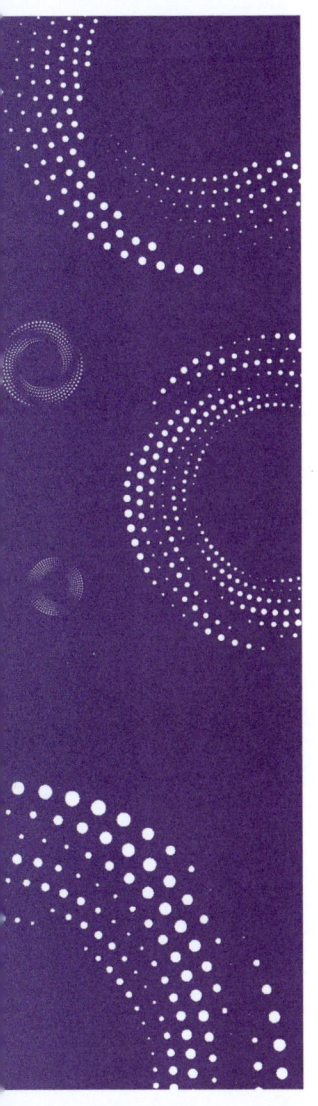

# Contents

# Introduction

Why do so many of us find it hard to get through the day without a clawing sense of anxiety? From disturbing news reports to toxic social media arguments, the faster pace of life after the start of the Information Age seems geared toward making us all more anxious and stressed. This guide is packed full of friendly advice to help you take control of your life and calm those oppressive feelings of worry and strife. It offers tips and tricks to soothe your nerves and help you develop a confident, calm personality that others will respect and respond to. Whether at home, in the workplace or within your relationships with your loved ones, you can become self-assured and able to cope with whatever life throws at you. Following the philosophies the book offers will enable you to communicate effectively with others, deal with demanding situations, and retain your equilibrium. By learning these skills you will strengthen your ability to respond well to unexpected challenges, and remain positive and relaxed.

Empowerment is at the heart of living a life free of anxiety. Life is a treasure chest of wonders and delights, and this little book wwill show you how to claim your fair share of it.

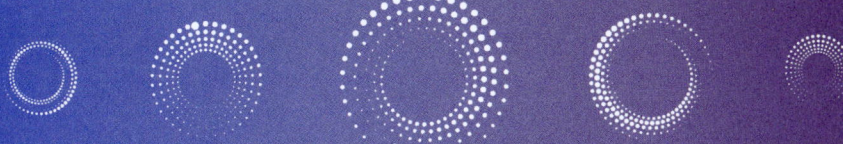

# What is Anxiety?

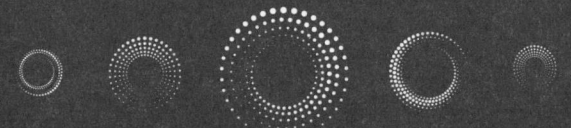

How do we define
anxiety, and what
makes it so important
in determining
how we cope in our
daily lives?

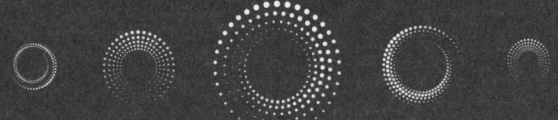

Our thoughts impact how we feel about the world. When we become anxious, we believe what are likely to be untrue thoughts and get stressed.

Serenity is simply finding the most direct path to your true self.

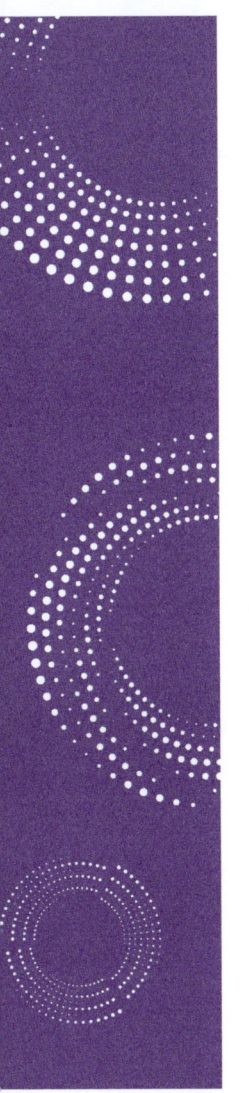

Knowing what is best for you, and how to achieve it, is the essence of empowering yourself.

A ship is safe in the harbour but that is not what ships are for.

*Albert J. Nimeth*

11

I think knowing what you cannot do is more important than knowing what you can.
*Lucille Ball*

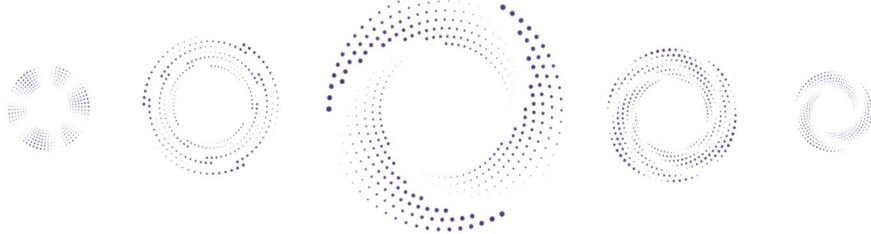

Each of us has a thousand potential selves that we could become. Contentment is making sure the right one wins out.

To feel free from intrusive thoughts, try this technique. Write out all your concerns and then cross them out, one by one.

Often physical exertion energizes rather than drains us. Similarly, when you're feeling anxious, it can be calming to do exercise. You get out of your head and into your body.

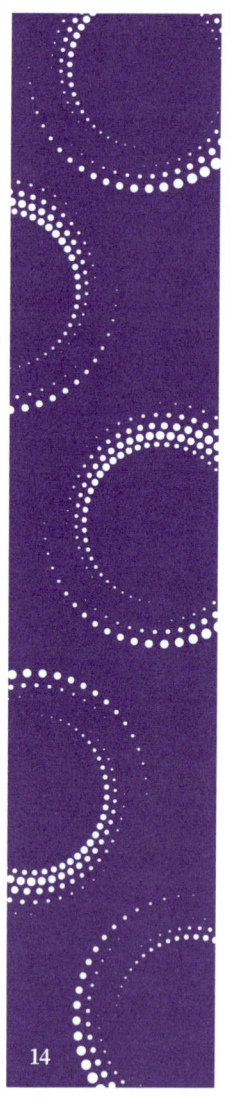

Do you feel weak? Good news: recognizing the need to empower yourself is half the battle. Those who think they are perfect, are conceited not empowered.

Everyone has to start their journey of self-discovery somewhere, so why not start yours here, and now?

No matter how empowered you become, there is always more left in the tank.

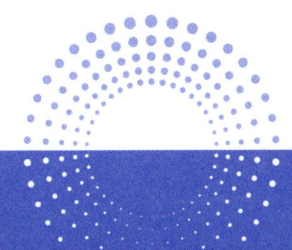

It is often easier to comfort others than it is to comfort ourselves, because we find it easier to see clearly what it is that others need. The difficult part of self-soothing is looking honestly into ourselves and our needs.

One of the prerequisites of a calm mind is an open one.

**Every moment is a fresh beginning.**
*T. S. Eliot*

Empowerment is nothing unless it results in action.

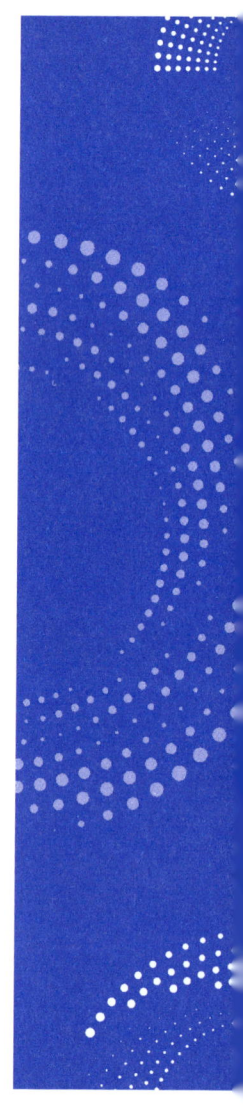

At the core of self-knowledge lies humility, not arrogance.

Contentment radiates outwards, so that contented people delight and make happy all those that they come into contact with.

A key aspect of empowering ourselves away from anxiety is knowing when to exercise our power and when to hold fire.

It takes just the right amount of self-belief and just the right amount of self-doubt to create self-empowerment.

The beauty of life is, while we cannot undo what is done, we can see it, understand it, learn from it and change. So that every new moment is spent not in regret, guilt, fear or anger, but in wisdom, understanding and love.

*Jennifer Edwards*

To have a dream, and live it – that is joy.

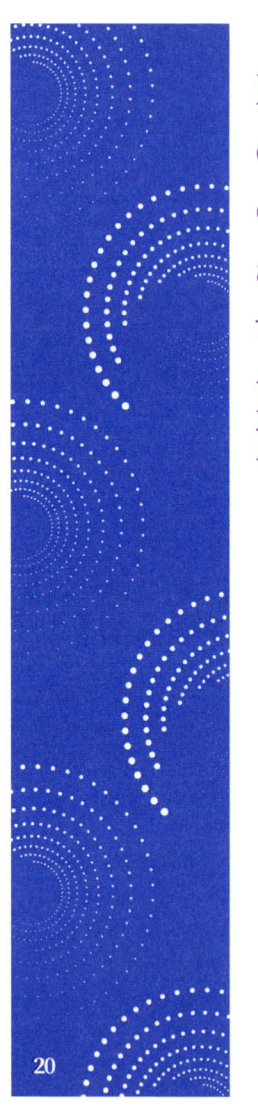

Many people confuse self-empowerment with having power over others. The trappings of power are insubstantial things that could be taken from you in a moment; inner power is far more potent because it belongs to you, and to you alone.

Nothing in life is to be feared. It is only to be understood.
*Marie Curie*

The easiest way to develop a resilient approach to life is to be generous towards others. If you can interpret actions in a kinder way, it will help you stay calm.

When all else fails, take a hot bath and let the water take away your worries.

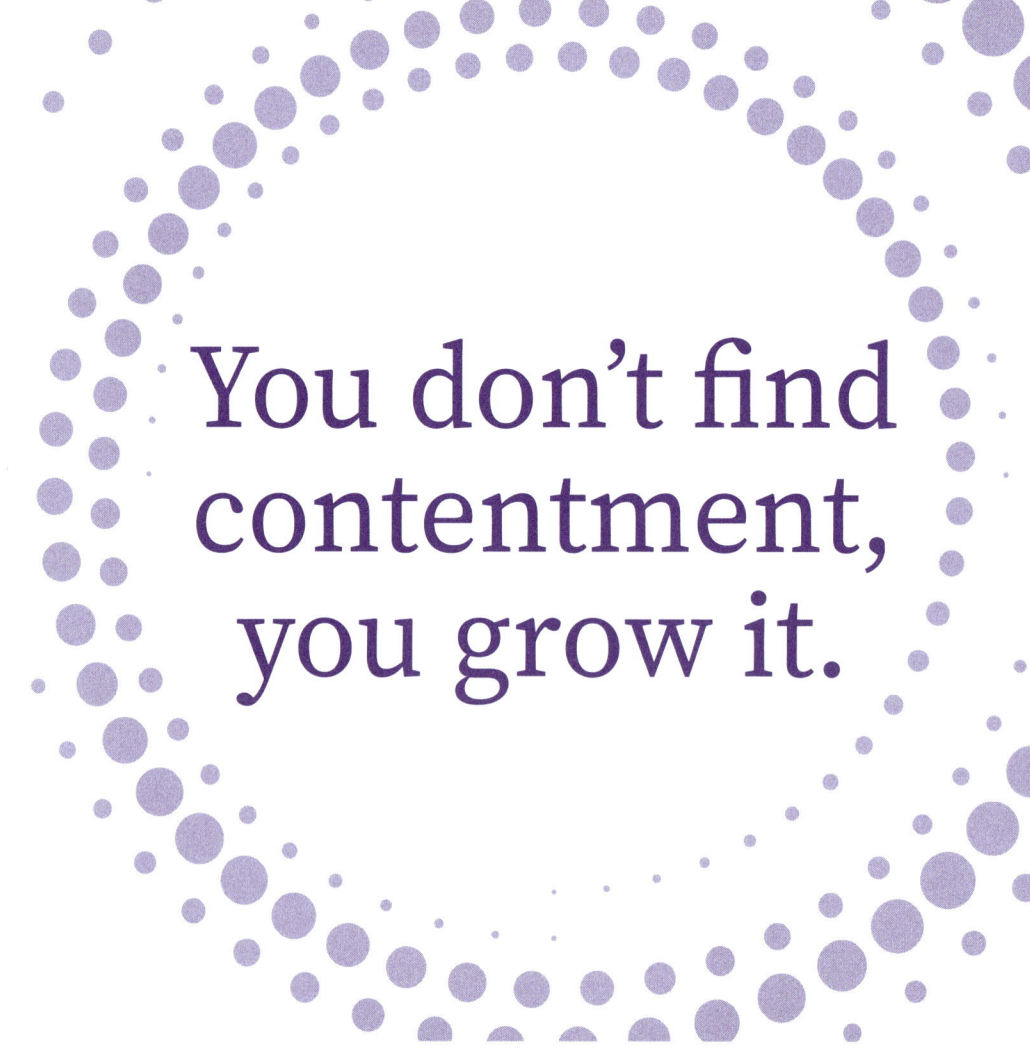

You don't find contentment, you grow it.

Go your own way.
Light your own path.
Be your own guide.

**Empowerment is not about always feeling strong. It is about how you respond when you are feeling weak.**

Empowerment is the inner fortress which protects you from day-to-day setbacks.

# To admit you don't know everything is the first step on the road to wisdom.

Power is only true power when you own it, rather than renting it. And the only power you ever truly own is the power of the self.

All the art of living lies in a fine mingling of letting go and holding on.
*Havelock Ellis*

A belief is only a thought you continue to think. A belief is nothing more than a chronic pattern of thought, and you have the ability – if you try even a little bit – to begin a new pattern, to tell a new story, to achieve a different vibration, to change your point of attraction.

*Abraham Hicks*

Empowerment is when you stop just going through life, and start growing through life instead.

It is harder for anxiety to take hold when you are operating at your full potential.

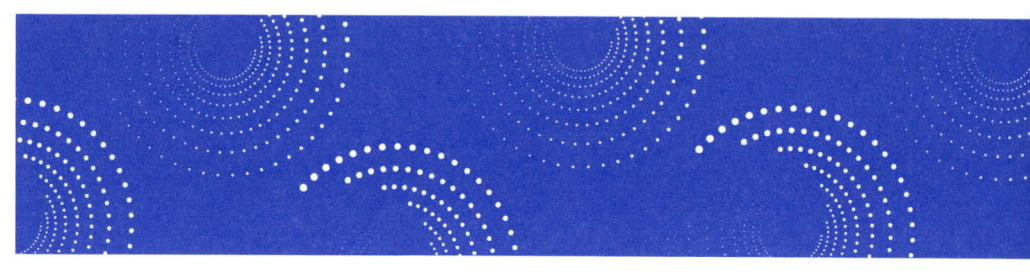

Life and change are the same things. When you embrace change, you embrace life.

We are the sum total of our choices. Empowerment means choosing wisely.

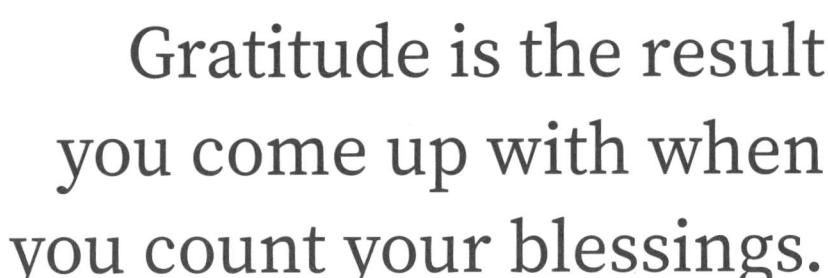

Gratitude is the result you come up with when you count your blessings.

There is no magic recipe for equilibrium, but self-belief is always one of the ingredients.

**One does not discover new lands without consenting to lose sight of the shore for a very long time.**
*André Gide*

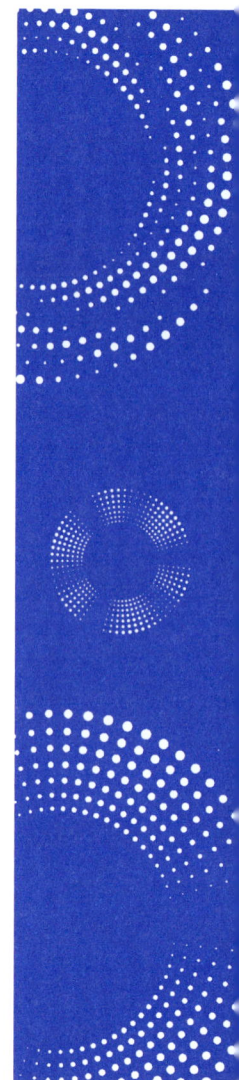

# Following in the footsteps of others will take you where they want to go, not where you want to go.

Empowerment is realizing that wanting what you get is more important than getting what you want.

**The meaning of life is to find your gift, the purpose of life is to give it away.**
*Joy J. Golliver*

Doubt builds walls to block our progress; empowerment tunnels under them.

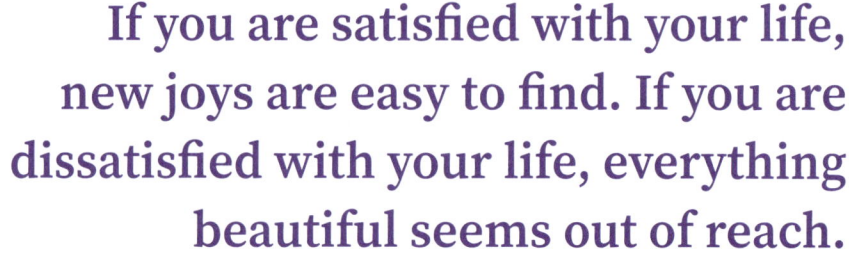

If you are satisfied with your life, new joys are easy to find. If you are dissatisfied with your life, everything beautiful seems out of reach.

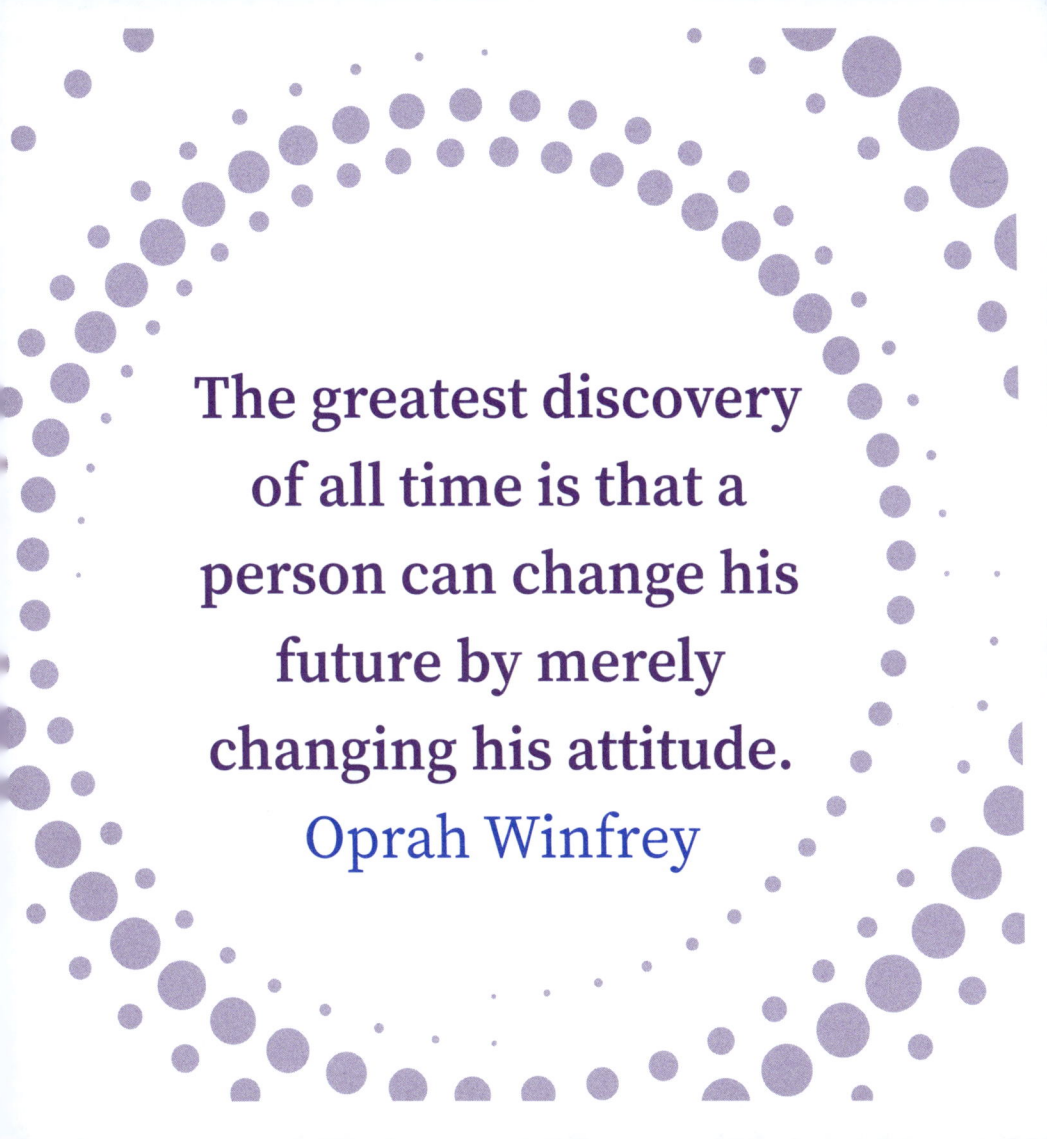

The greatest discovery
of all time is that a
person can change his
future by merely
changing his attitude.
Oprah Winfrey

In the dead of winter, the simple act of believing in spring is a type of empowerment.

**Fear makes us want to look down at how far we might fall; empowerment turns its face to the stars and just climbs.**

Empowerment is a tiny act of faith that can make all the difference to your life: all that you have to believe is that you have a talent for something. You must, however, believe that tiny fact with all your being.

**Nobody knows what tomorrow will bring, which is why the wise believe in today.**

When you are content to be simply yourself and don't compare or compete, everybody will respect you.
*Lao Tzu*

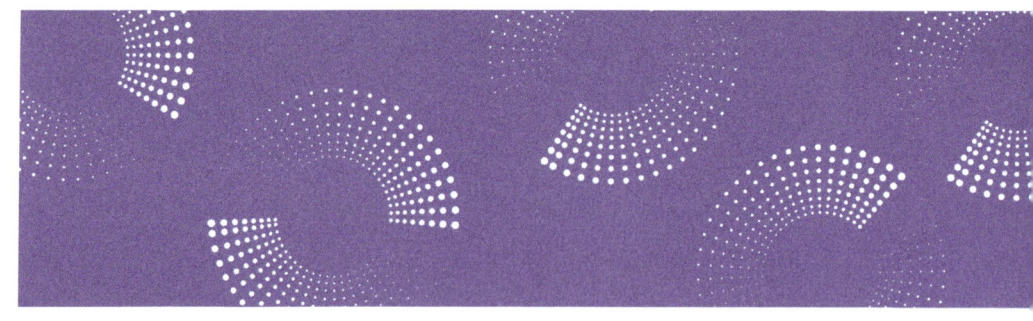

What's the worst that can happen?
How likely is it to come to pass? It is
rarely ever as bad as we think it is.

**Resilient people
make new resolutions
every day, not once a year.**

When your heart begins to lead you somewhere, push it in that direction with all your strength.

Change will not come if we wait for some other person or some other time. We are the ones we've been waiting for. We are the change that we seek.

*Barack Obama*

There are so many worthwhile things to do each and every day. Happiness is working out which of them means most to you.

**Choose rather to be strong of soul than strong of body.**
*Pythagoras*

Celebrate your daily wins – even small ones. Being awake and dressed is sometimes enough.

**Don't run from sadness. Sit with it until it lessens its hold.**

Empowerment is to the soul what the acorn is to the oak tree.

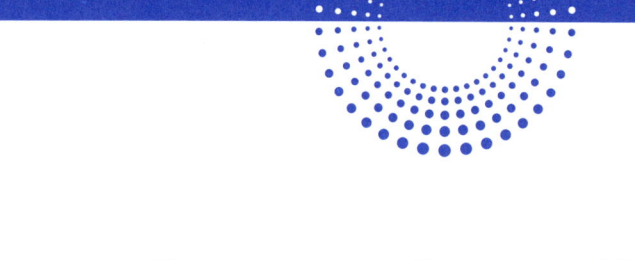

The rest of your life begins every day. Don't waste it. Begin your journey to joy today.

Life is not something that just happens to you. You have control and create the life you want for yourself with daily decisions.

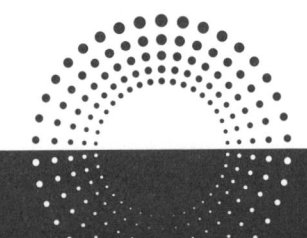

Being silent isn't being strong, it's being a victim.

*Jane Powell*

**Contentment is a factory that produces positivity from the raw material of daily life.**

The relaxed person is constantly seeking new experiences and visiting new places.

**Where there is no struggle, there is no strength.**
*Oprah Winfrey*

If negativity does not
exist in your world,
empowerment
is already in your heart.

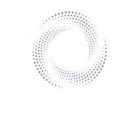

We know what we are,
but not what we may be.

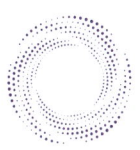

*William Shakespeare*

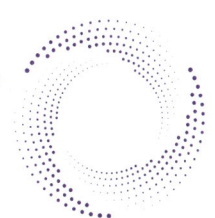

# Curiosity
# is enthusiasm
# in action.

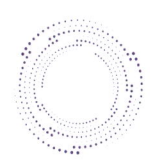

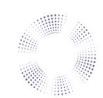

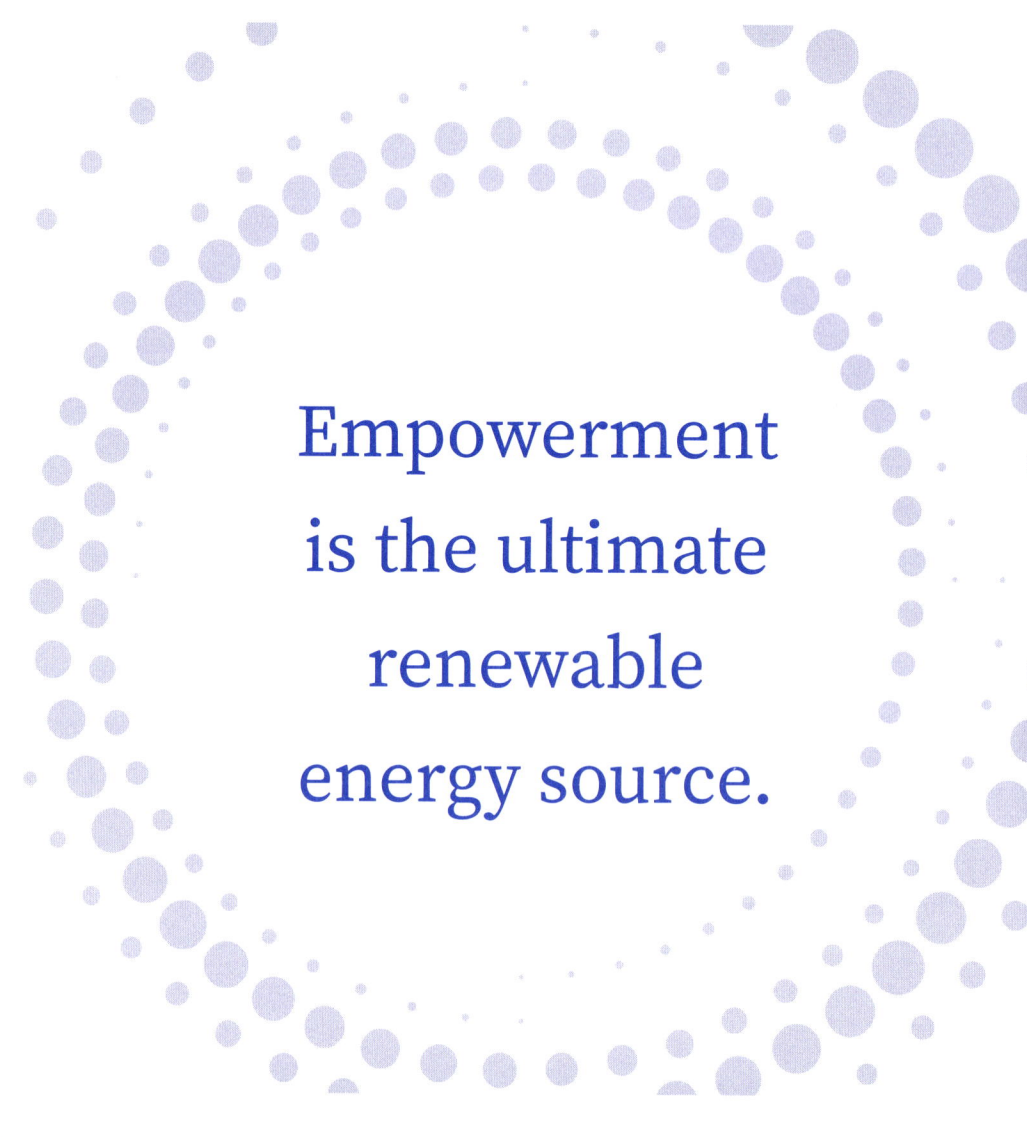

Empowerment
is the ultimate
renewable
energy source.

Praise and criticism are both grist to the mill for the resolved person.

Real knowledge is to know the extent of one's ignorance.
*Confucius*

You can talk yourself out of anxiety. It is a case of thinking out what you're anxious about and robustly meeting each fear with a rational answer.

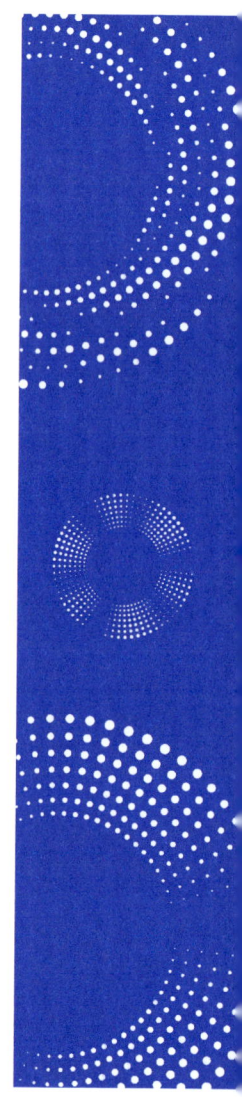

Ninety per cent of good living is rolling your sleeves up and getting stuck in.

Empowerment is unstoppable, because it constantly renews itself.

The resilient person believes that the whole world is conspiring to help them achieve their goals.

Flowers need both sun and rain in order to grow, and we need failure in order to appreciate success.

Just a small step of self-belief each day will support your love of the world.

Sometimes our own worst enemy lives between our ears: to cope with anxiety you must first make friends with yourself.

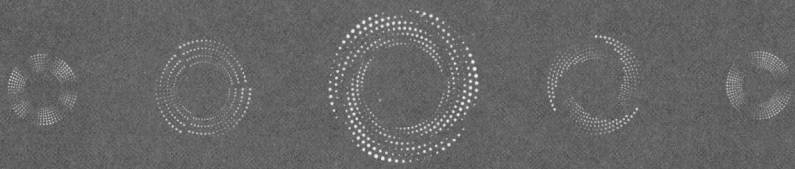

Ideals are like stars; you will not succeed in touching them with your hands. But like the seafaring man on the desert of waters, you choose them as your guides, and following them you will reach your destiny.

*Carl Schurz*

**Stay as prepared as possible. If you fail to prepare then you are preparing to fail.**

You must be willing to risk losing in the short term in order to gain in the long term.

Life is full of hard knocks. It is empowerment that lifts you back onto your feet when you feel you can't get up.

An athlete cannot run with money in his pockets. He must run with hope in his heart and dreams in his head.
Emil Zátopek

Dreams are evidence that we are creatures who produce more meaning than we can ourselves understand.
*Mark Kingwell*

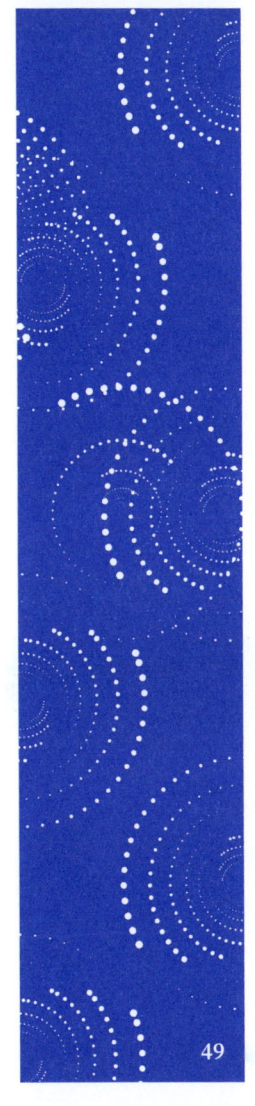

**Medals tarnish and trophies gather dust: serene people know that the true rewards are the ones you carry forever in your heart.**

The harder the struggle, the sweeter the victory.

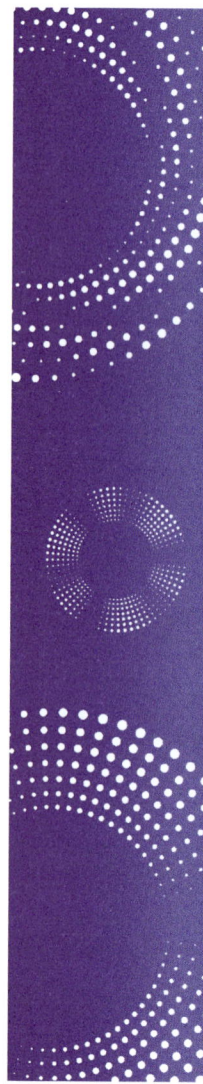

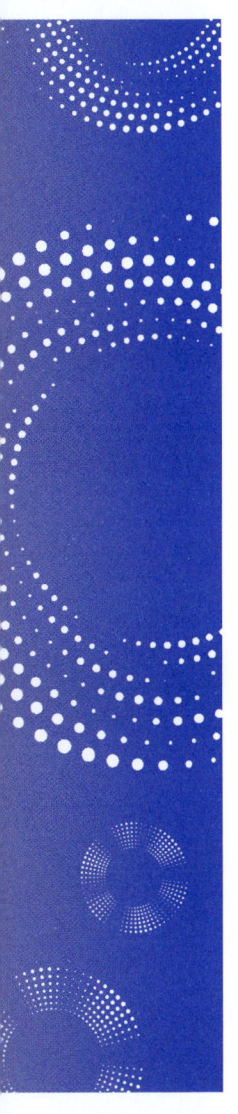

Equanimity makes little difference when the odds are in your favour; it is when the odds are against you that it becomes valuable.

**Age is no barrier. It's a limitation you put on your mind.**
*Jackie Joyner-Kersee*

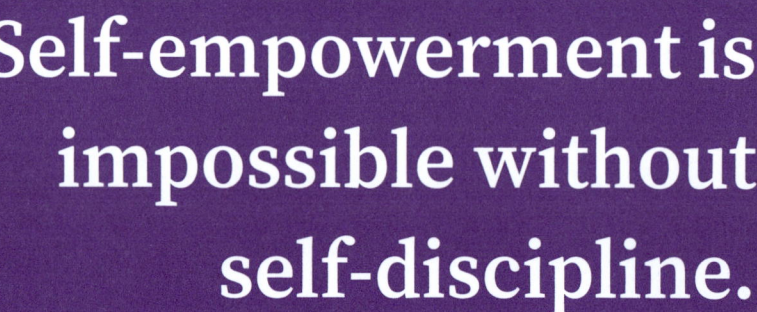

**Self-empowerment is impossible without self-discipline.**

Fear is the only motivation that some people know. Empowered people have a much stronger motivation: confidence.

Work hard, but know the value of play too – that's the secret to staying anxiety free.

Never be afraid to look or feel ridiculous. Vanity is the enemy of joy.

# Where are you going, if you aren't prepared to go all the way?

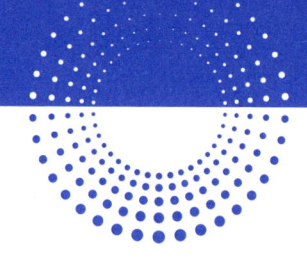

To become empowered you must first find your limits and then have the courage to go past them.

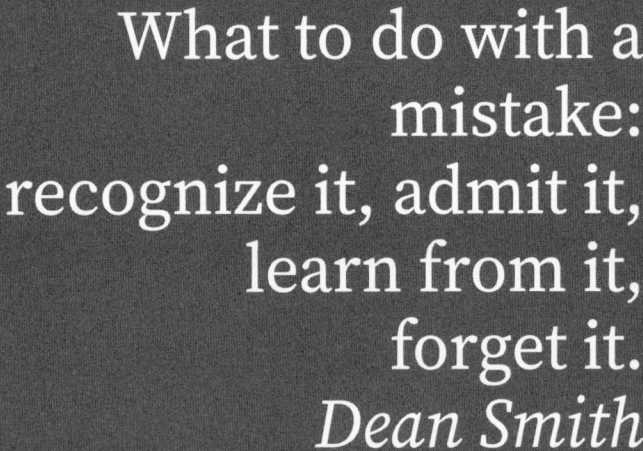

What to do with a mistake: recognize it, admit it, learn from it, forget it.
*Dean Smith*

You can't avoid fear, but you can train yourself not to let it cripple you. When you can continue with your day despite the fear, you will conquer it.

Often composure isn't a matter of finding the way – it's a matter of finding another way.

# The short-cut to a happier life is to just try things out.

Despair is a failure of imagination. Keep imagining a better outcome.

# All difficulties are temporary: only quitting lasts forever.

It's not the will to win that matters – everyone has that. It's the will to prepare to win that matters.
*Paul Bryant*

## Empowered people come in all shapes and sizes: the only size that matters is the size of your heart.

No matter how physically frail or unwell you are, no matter how young or how old, knowing how to relax can transform your life.

We do not ask for what useful purpose the birds do sing, for song is their pleasure since they were created for singing.
*Johannes Kepler*

Imagine what the world would look like if every person realized their full potential. You can do your bit towards making that dream come true by becoming empowered, and encouraging others to become empowered too.

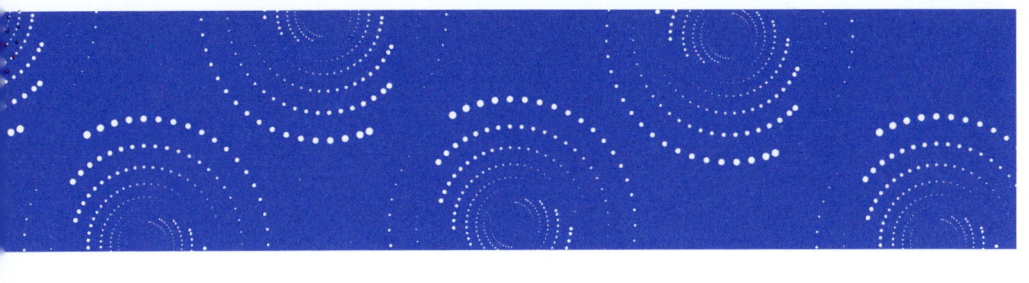

Nothing comes from nothing: happiness is born from a desire to change.

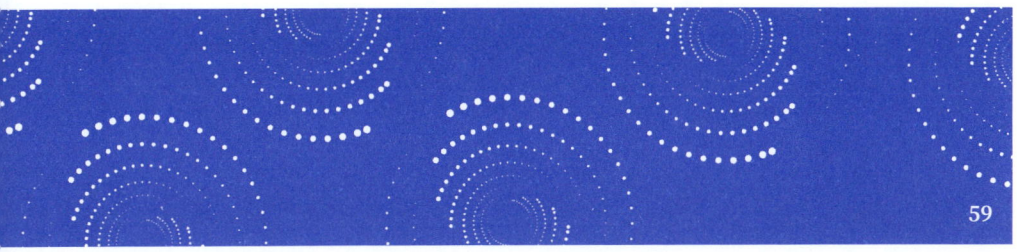

Empowerment is not the same as optimism: the empowered person is a realist, who acknowledges the difficulties of life but remains resolutely determined to overcome them.

Return to the breath whenever the world overwhelms you.

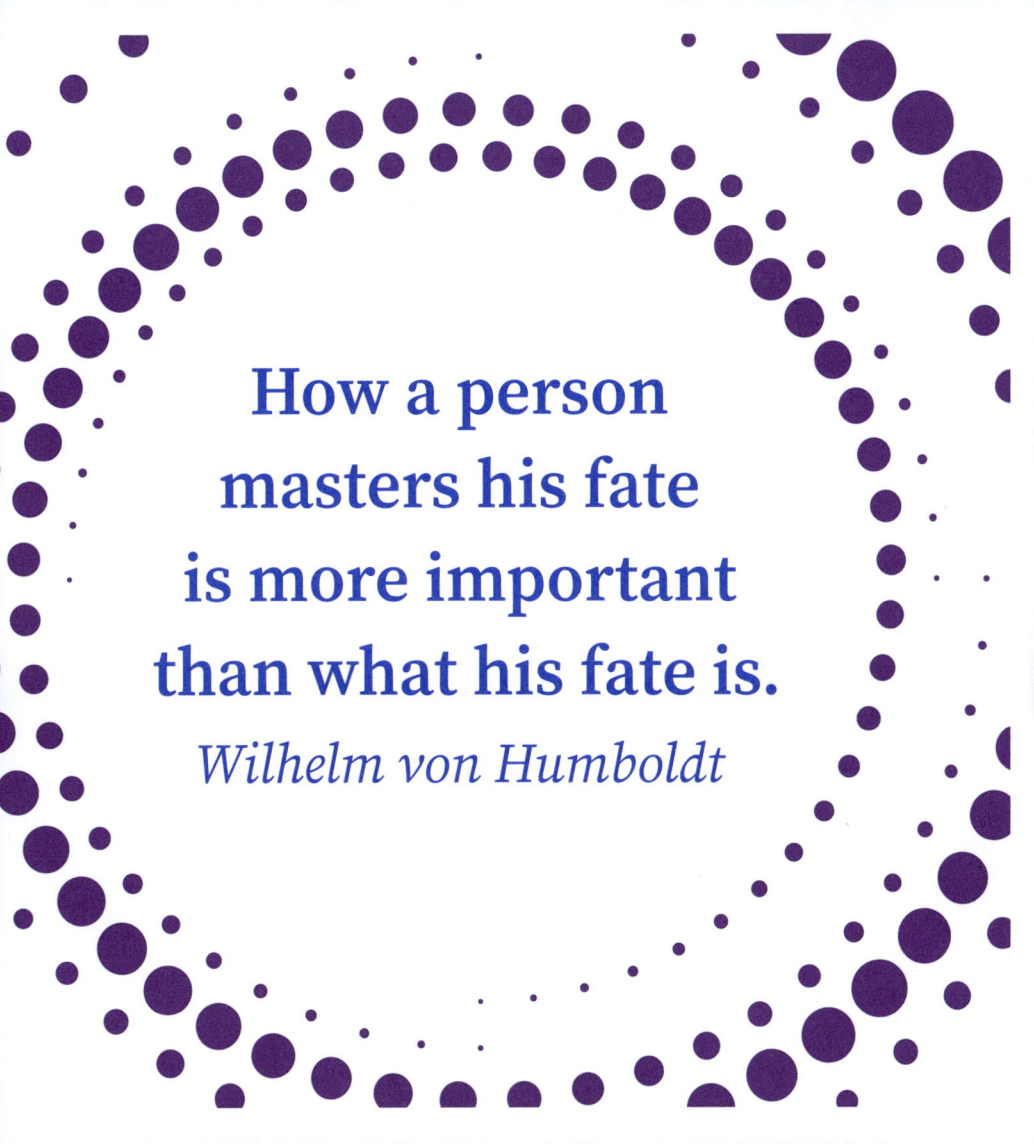

How a person
masters his fate
is more important
than what his fate is.
*Wilhelm von Humboldt*

You have had days without anxiety and you will have again. Remember that.

Simply copying what others do will never lead to happiness. You learn better by doing things yourself, and seeing what works best for you.

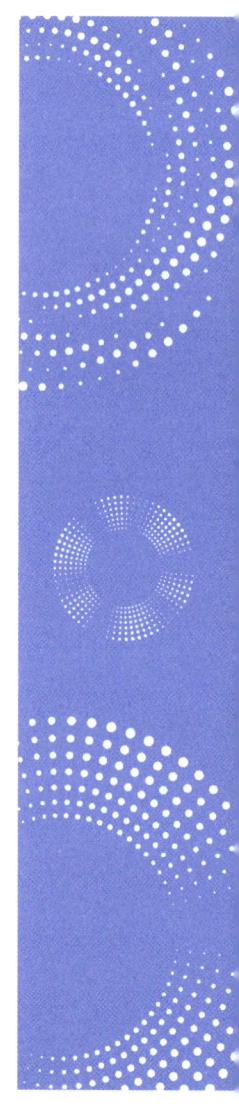

Anxiety tells you that you are alone, but this is simply not the case. Find your tribe; let them help.

We can be given power by others, but only we can empower ourselves.

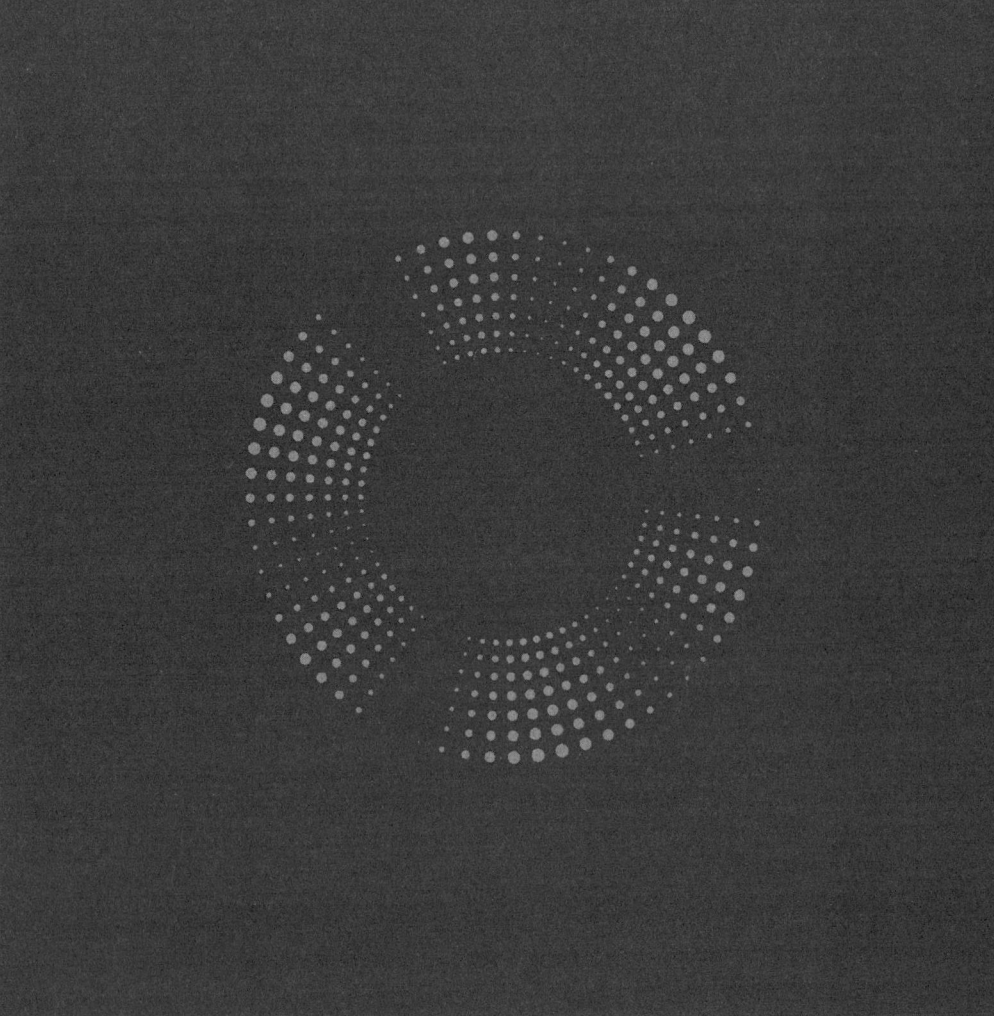

# Finding the Way

Some people seem to find it easy to remain calm and self-assured, while others suffer from doubt and anxiety. How do we learn to trust in our own judgement, and how can we project that new-found confidence effectively?

Go out of your way to spare the feelings of others, but never at the expense of telling the truth. In the end, remaining truthful will gain you the respect of others.

**A good traveller has no fixed plans, and is not intent on arriving.**
*Lao Tzu*

Keeping things in perspective can help to lessen anxiety. Remember that we can often unhelpfully catastrophize and it is always good to interrogate your assumptions about the world around you.

Share everything in your life with others. What you give will return to you a hundred times over.

Being firm does not mean being impolite: communicate your desires clearly, but always be polite, and don't forget to smile.

Whenever you can, take a moment to rebalance yourself. Close your eyes, take a deep breath, and remind yourself that you are capable of great things.

**Eat healthily, even if you are in a rush. A healthy body leads to a healthy mind.**

Nobody can go back
and start a new beginning,
but anyone can start today
and make a new ending.
*Maria Robinson*

**Whatever the present moment contains, accept it as if you had chosen it.**
*Eckhart Tolle*

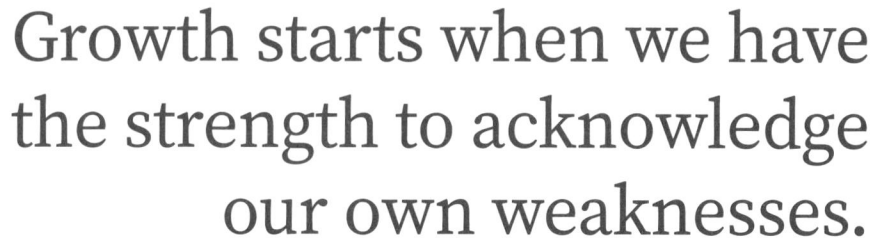

Growth starts when we have the strength to acknowledge our own weaknesses.

If you're in any doubt about what you are going to say, stay silent until you are sure. Nothing is more damaging than saying something you later regret.

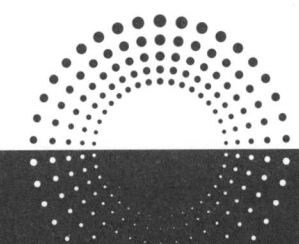

Remember that just because somebody throws you a problem, it doesn't mean that you have to catch it.

The more you dwell on what you don't have, the more you get what you don't want.

Take plenty of exercise. You will feel as though you have more energy, and others will feel that energy radiating from you.

Whatever you think, you eventually become – so think positively.

The way to predict the future is to create it yourself.

Keep a list of things
you want to achieve each
day, and tackle the items on
the list one by one. Focusing
on the task in hand is the
way to get things done.

If you believe in yourself
you can achieve anything,
but if you doubt yourself you
can achieve nothing.

I keep the telephone of my mind open to peace, harmony, health, love, and abundance. Then, whenever doubt, anxiety, or fear try to call me, they will keep getting a busy signal – and soon they'll forget my number.

*Edith Armstrong*

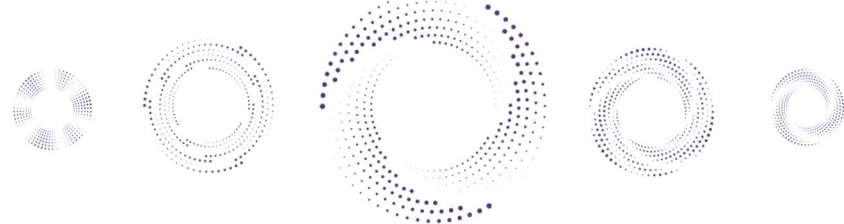

Sometimes sitting with an uncomfortable emotion can be the only thing to be done.

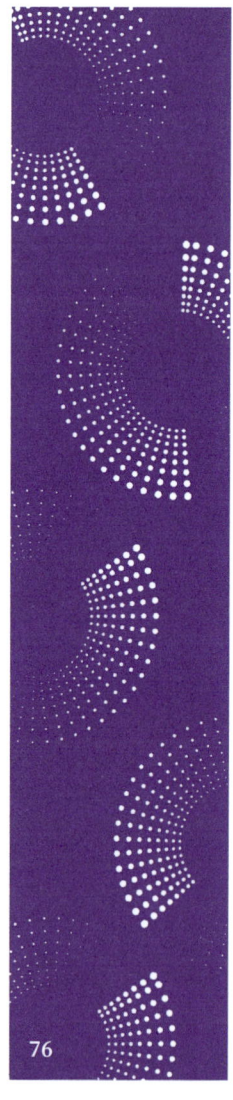

Celebrate your own uniqueness. Nobody who has ever lived has been quite the same as you are.

Great minds discuss ideas. Average minds discuss events. Small minds discuss people.
*Eleanor Roosevelt*

The reason distractions are so dangerous is because deep down we love them. Accept this and ensure that you keep your 'distraction time' separate from your working time.

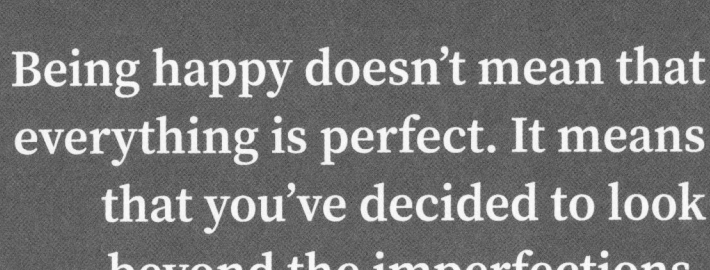

Being happy doesn't mean that everything is perfect. It means that you've decided to look beyond the imperfections.

If you look into your own heart,
and you find nothing wrong there,
what is there to worry about?
What is there to fear?
*Confucius*

Start by establishing a goal,
break that goal down into
a series of milestones, and
then list the tasks you need
to complete to get to the
first milestone. By working
methodically through all the
tasks, you will eventually
arrive at your goal.

# To improve you must learn, and to learn you must recognize that you don't know everything.

Empowered people sometimes have to assert themselves in order to get where they want to go – but they also know that conflict should be avoided whenever possible. Learning the art of diplomacy is vital if you want to stay in control.

Talents are best nurtured in solitude, but character is best formed in the stormy billows of the world.
*Goethe*

Lift yourself up, don't pull yourself down.

Reward yourself: don't wait for others to praise you – sometimes you need to pat your own back.

People will find it easier to accept criticism from you if you acknowledge their strengths first.

Remember to enjoy your successes: sometimes we are so focused on the next problem we forget to celebrate our triumphs.

If you only do what you've always done, you'll only get what you've always had.

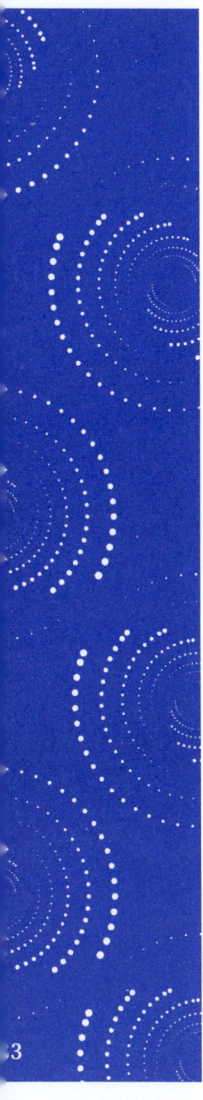

To be ambitious is no bad thing, but if you set your expectations of yourself unrealistically high then you will doom yourself to forever fall short.

---

Nobody would exhaust themselves climbing mountains if the view didn't make it worthwhile. Visualize what your life will be like when you achieve your goal, and use that to motivate you when the mountain seems especially steep.

It is you that decides whether or not you will be happy, not the events that happen to you.

—————————————————○

**Learn to accept praise. Don't tell those who praise you they are wrong: just say thanks and you'll both feel better.**

—————————————————○

The difference between a wish and a goal is a plan.

Smell is a potent wizard that transports you across thousands of miles and all the years you have lived. *Helen Keller*

Routine can crush your enthusiasm without you even noticing it. Don't just ask yourself how you can do things better, ask yourself how you can do things differently. Often doing something differently results in you doing it better, too.

What you think
of yourself is far
more important
than what others
think of you.

Forget yesterday and do not worry about tomorrow, just focus on being happy today.

First simplify your life: the essential things will be easier to find if they are not hidden by unnecessary clutter.

Chart your own course, even if others warn you of strong headwinds.

**Sitting quietly, doing nothing, spring comes, and the grass grows by itself.**

*Zen proverb*

---

Prioritize work that must be done over work that you could have done.

Remember that what you see as a flaw might be exactly what somebody else sees as a strength.

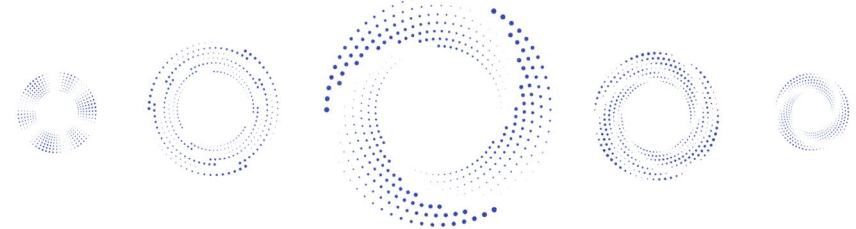

**To know yet to think that one does not know is best; not to know yet to think that one knows will lead to difficulty.**

*Lao Tzu*

Live as if you have already accomplished everything you would like to achieve. Treat everything from here on as icing on the cake.

You cannot become empowered and remain in your comfort zone at the same time. That doesn't mean you have to dismantle your comfort zone – you just need to extend it bit by bit until your comfort zone is the whole world.

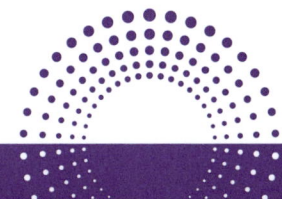

Aim high! The future you see is the person you will be.

*Jim Cathcart*

Trying to multi-task often results in you doing everything badly. Do the important things well, and the rest will take care of itself.

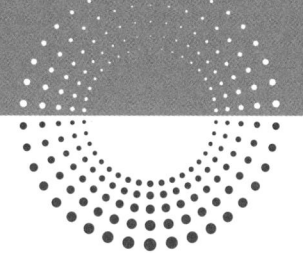

There's more than one way of skinning a cat, but before you think of a new way, ask yourself, 'What am I going to do with a cat's skin anyway?'

Sometimes we expend more energy on running away from a challenge than we would have spent if we had just stood our ground and tackled it head on.

If you celebrate, things to celebrate will come your way.

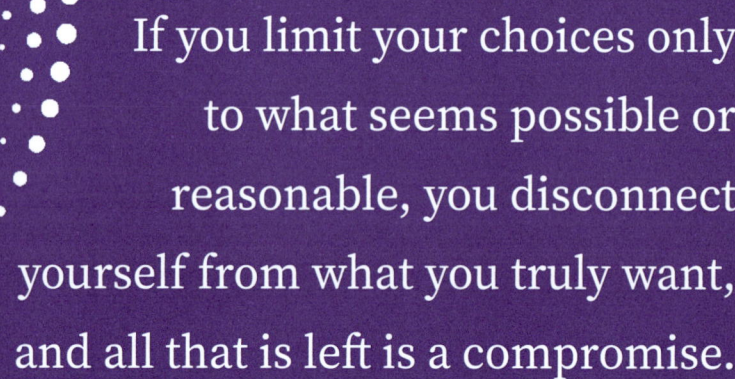

If you limit your choices only to what seems possible or reasonable, you disconnect yourself from what you truly want, and all that is left is a compromise.

*Robert Fritz*

All the fear we feel we create ourselves: if you list your fears and learn to look at them objectively you will find most of them disappear.

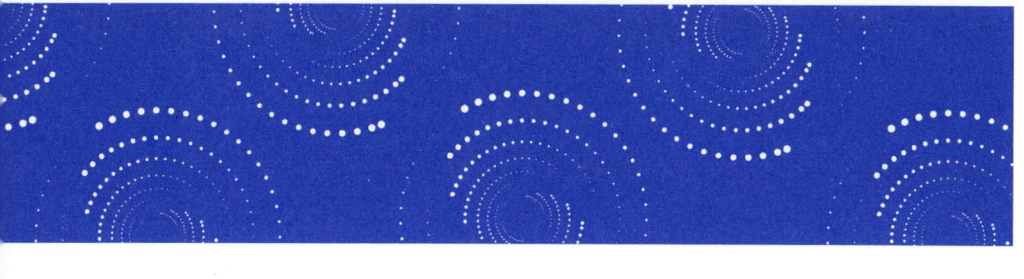

Nothing is destined for you; nothing good, nothing bad. You become the person you decide to be.

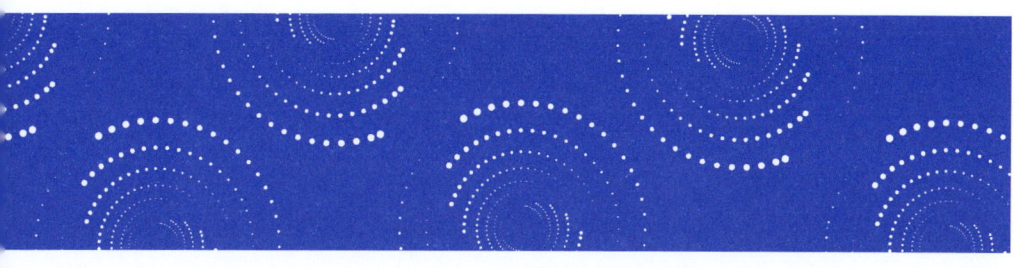

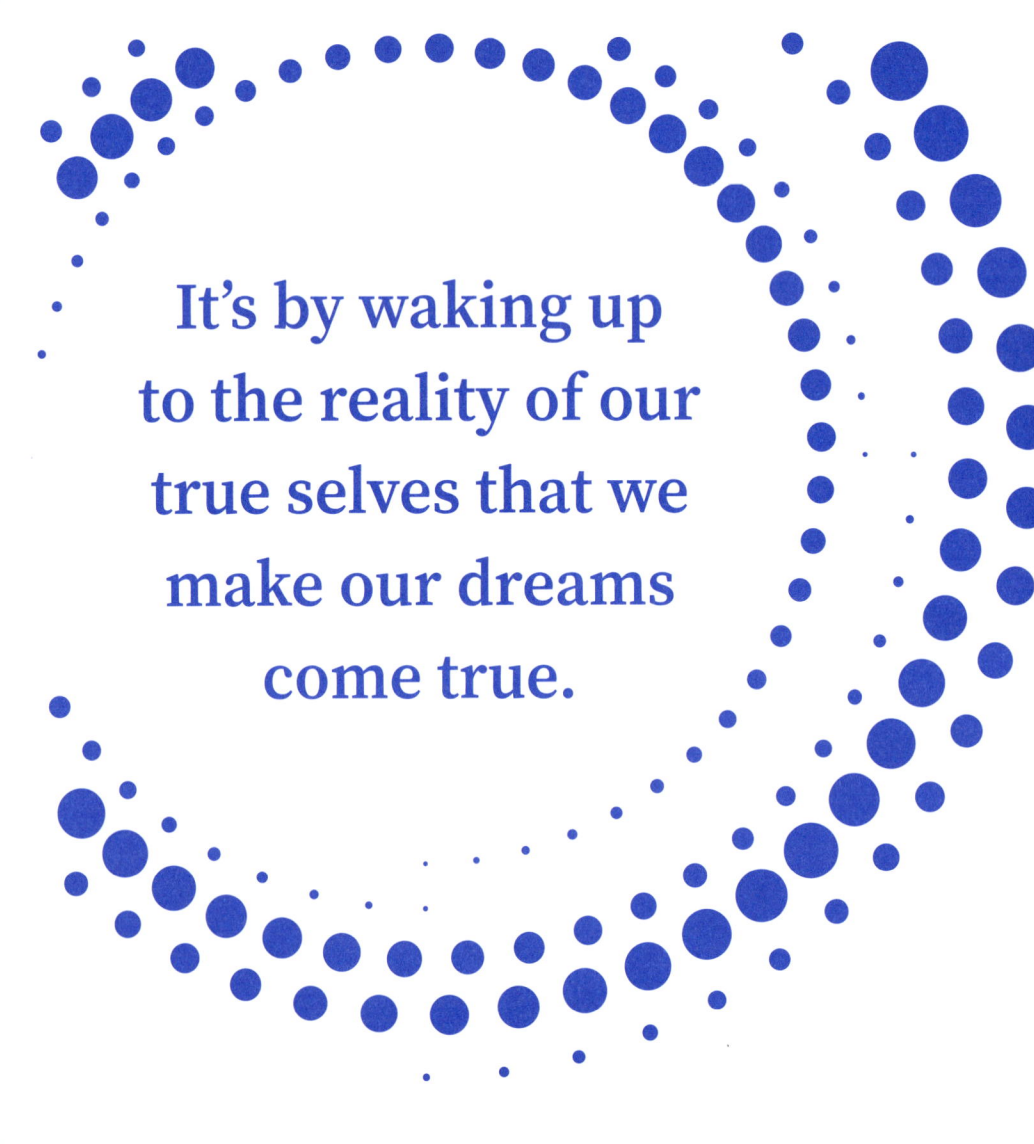

It's by waking up
to the reality of our
true selves that we
make our dreams
come true.

It is necessary to the happiness of
man that he be mentally faithful to
himself. Infidelity does not consist
in believing, or in disbelieving, it
consists in professing to believe
what he does not believe.

*Thomas Paine*

List the things you know you need to
do but don't really want to do. Tackle
the list one by one. We all tend to be
guilty of putting difficult things off, but
those who only ever do what they want
to do never grow to their full potential.

Going with the flow is all too easy, but you end up wherever the flow takes you, not where you really want to go.

There is no easier way to create calm than to notice what works, and then repeat it.

Birds use the air currents to help their flight; in the same way, the resilient person learns to constantly adjust their balance in the face of each day's events.

Sooner or later, moving in a straight line always takes you to an immovable obstacle. Be pragmatic, not dogmatic, in order to keep to your true path.

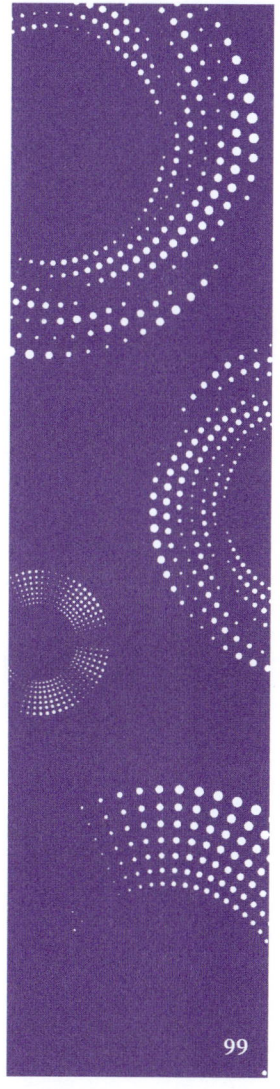

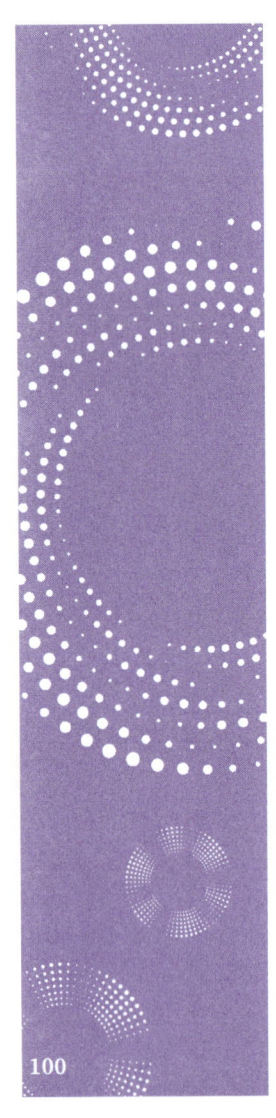

# Get mad, then get over it.
## *Colin Powell*

We all have weak points, and most of us tend to shy away from situations that will expose them. To become empowered, however, you must work on your weak points – and that means embracing situations that you know are going to be challenging for you.

Moments spent waiting
are moments wasted.

**Talk face to face whenever
you can. Email is great for
information, but lousy for
forming relationships and
having conversations.**

Don't ask yourself what the world needs,
ask yourself what makes you come alive.
And then go and do that. Because what the
world needs is people who are alive.

*Howard Thurman*

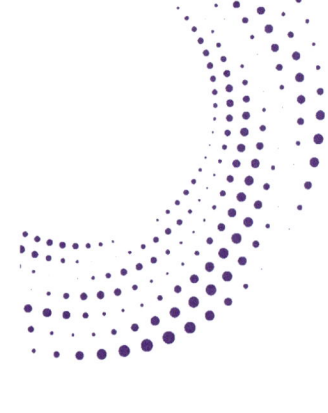

What's on the inside is more important than what's on the outside, but sometimes dressing to impress can give you that little extra boost of confidence you need to dazzle the world.

If you don't let go of the past you may well trip over something that is behind you.

The beautiful thing about learning is that nobody can take that away from you.
*B.B. King*

Start thinking of yourself as a success and it will be a great deal easier to become a success.

**Whom do you admire? When you're feeling anxious, ask yourself what your role model would do in your situation.**

Don't duck responsibility, grab it with both hands – even if doing so scares you. In the end, if you run away from responsibility you run away from opportunity too.

Be careful what you water your dreams with. Water them with worry and fear and you will produce weeds that choke the life from your dream. Water them with optimism and solutions and you will cultivate success.
*Lao Tzu*

———————————————————○

**Learn something new every day. It doesn't matter if it is a new fact, a new word or a new lesson from life; the important thing is to constantly learn and constantly improve.**

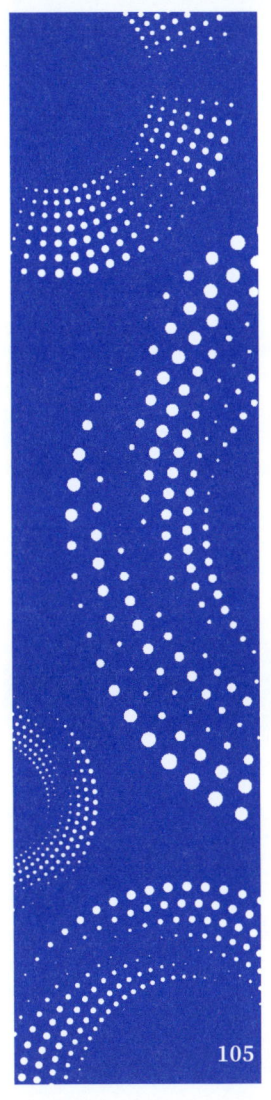

We all have an inner voice that casts doubts on our ability to achieve our dreams. Learn to recognize that voice, so that you can silence it or drown it out with a stronger inner voice.

What you see will depend largely on what you look for.

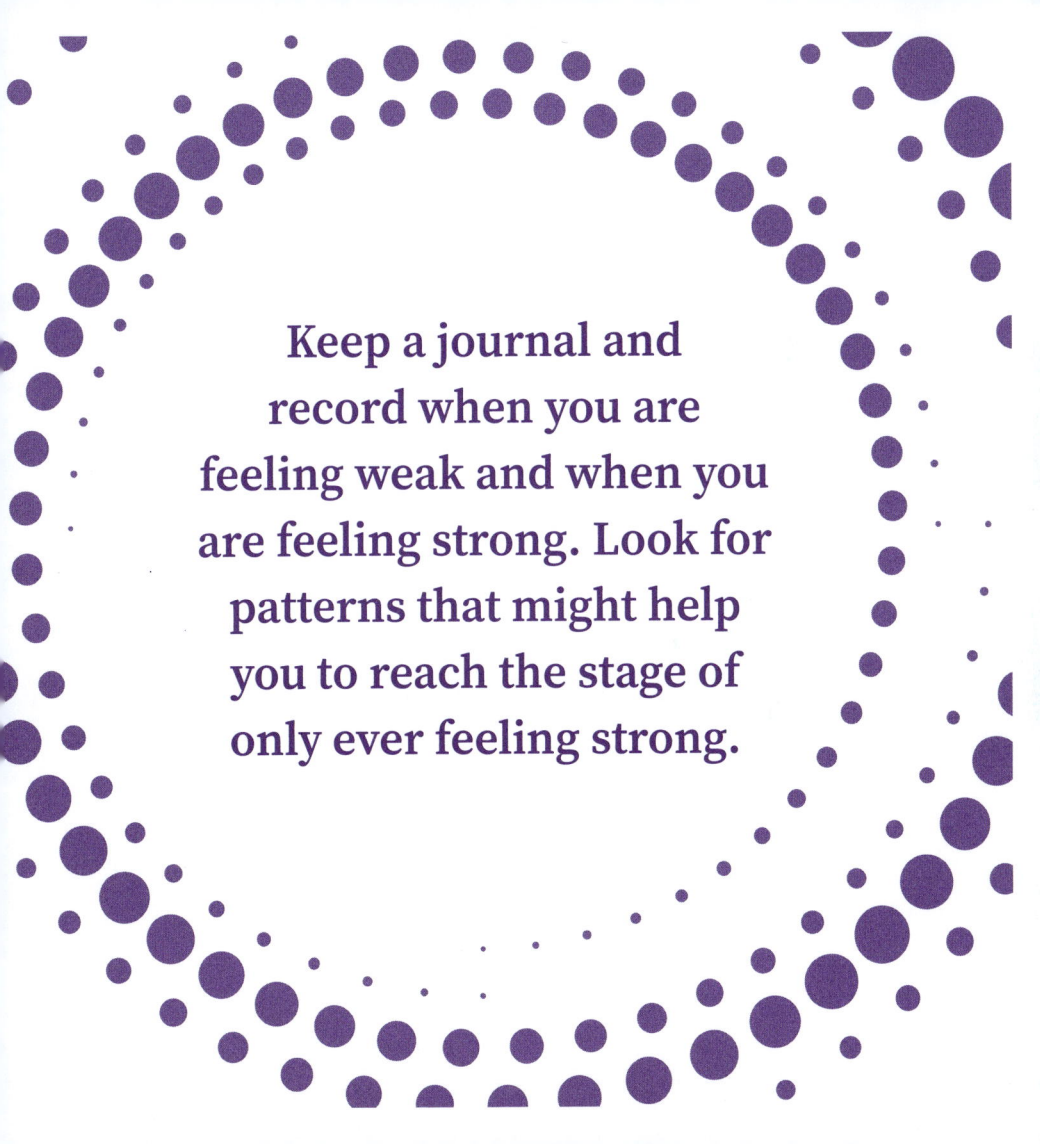

Keep a journal and record when you are feeling weak and when you are feeling strong. Look for patterns that might help you to reach the stage of only ever feeling strong.

If you pursue money and fame then you walk on a road without end, as you will never find enough of either. If you pursue only happiness then you will find it easily, as even a small amount goes a long way.

**Be kind whenever possible. And remember: it is always possible.**

You are braver than you believe, stronger than you seem, and smarter than you think.
*A.A. Milne*

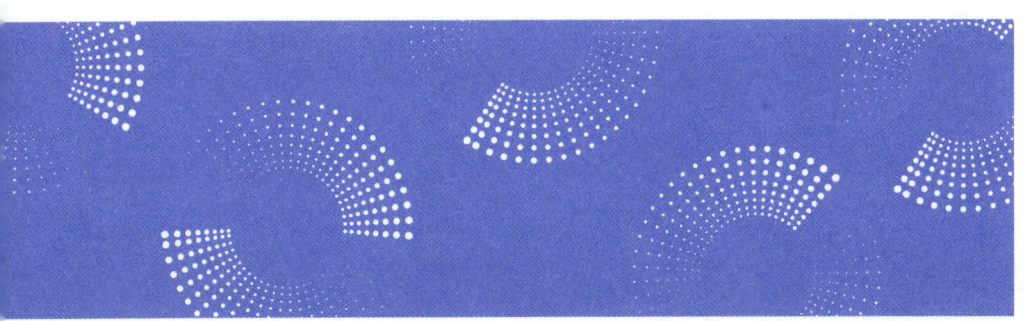

Ask new questions of yourself each and every day. The right answers are a good deal less important than the right questions.

Do you really need all that you currently possess? Throwing something out can often be an intensely liberating experience.

Research suggests that just by thinking happy thoughts we become happier. The same is true with serenity: begin to believe that you are calm and you will instantly feel more relaxed.

Stop working at least an hour before you go to bed. Your mind needs time to wind down, and you will feel better if you have had a good night's sleep.

---

# Tell yourself this each morning: no matter what obstacles I encounter today, I will overcome them with renewed inner strength.

---

The greatest mistake you can make in life is to be continually fearing you will make one.
*Elbert Hubbard*

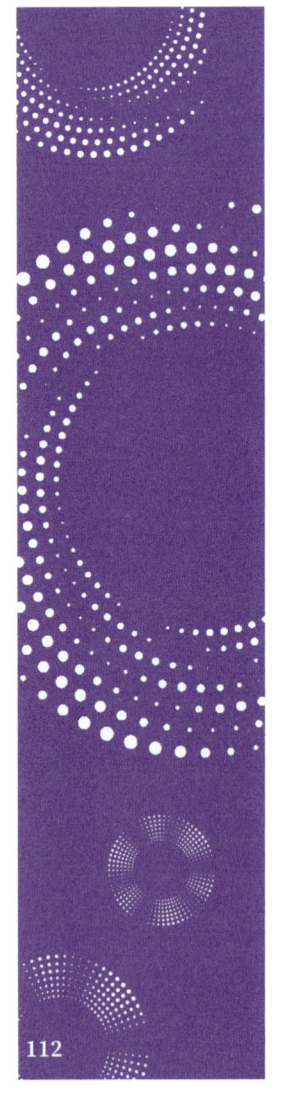

Maintaining a sense of humour is the most empowering thing that any of us can do.

In order to grow, it is more important to break bad habits than to develop good habits.

Learn to view advertisements with scepticism: they often sell us the idea that we are weak, in order to suggest that purchasing a certain product will make us feel more confident.

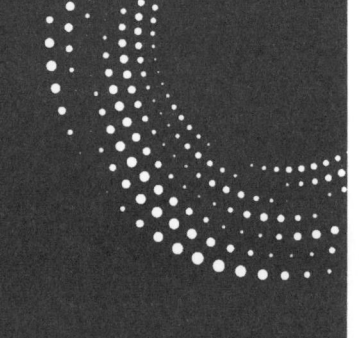

Visualize where you would most like to be tomorrow. We always end up where our thoughts lead us.

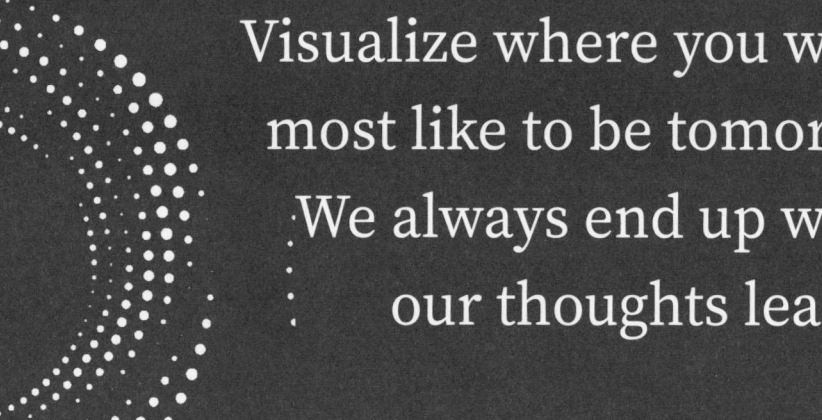

He who asks is a fool for five minutes, but he who does not ask remains a fool forever.

*Chinese proverb*

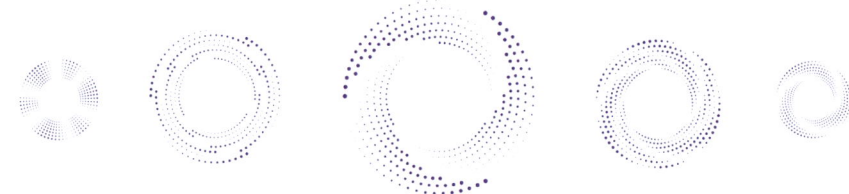

**Helping others is noble and kind, but make sure you are not subconsciously surrounding yourself with people whose needs are dragging you down.**

We don't get to choose everything that happens to us, but we do get to decide which memories we will focus on. Make sure you remember your past triumphs, not your past disasters.

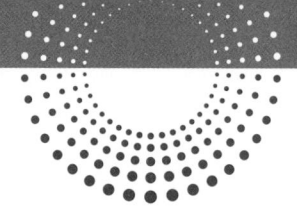

Only open your mouth to inform others, not to make yourself look smart.

**Sometimes you have to change paths many times in order to reach your destination.**

The world is a mirror. If you want the world to look kindly upon you, you have to look kindly upon it first.

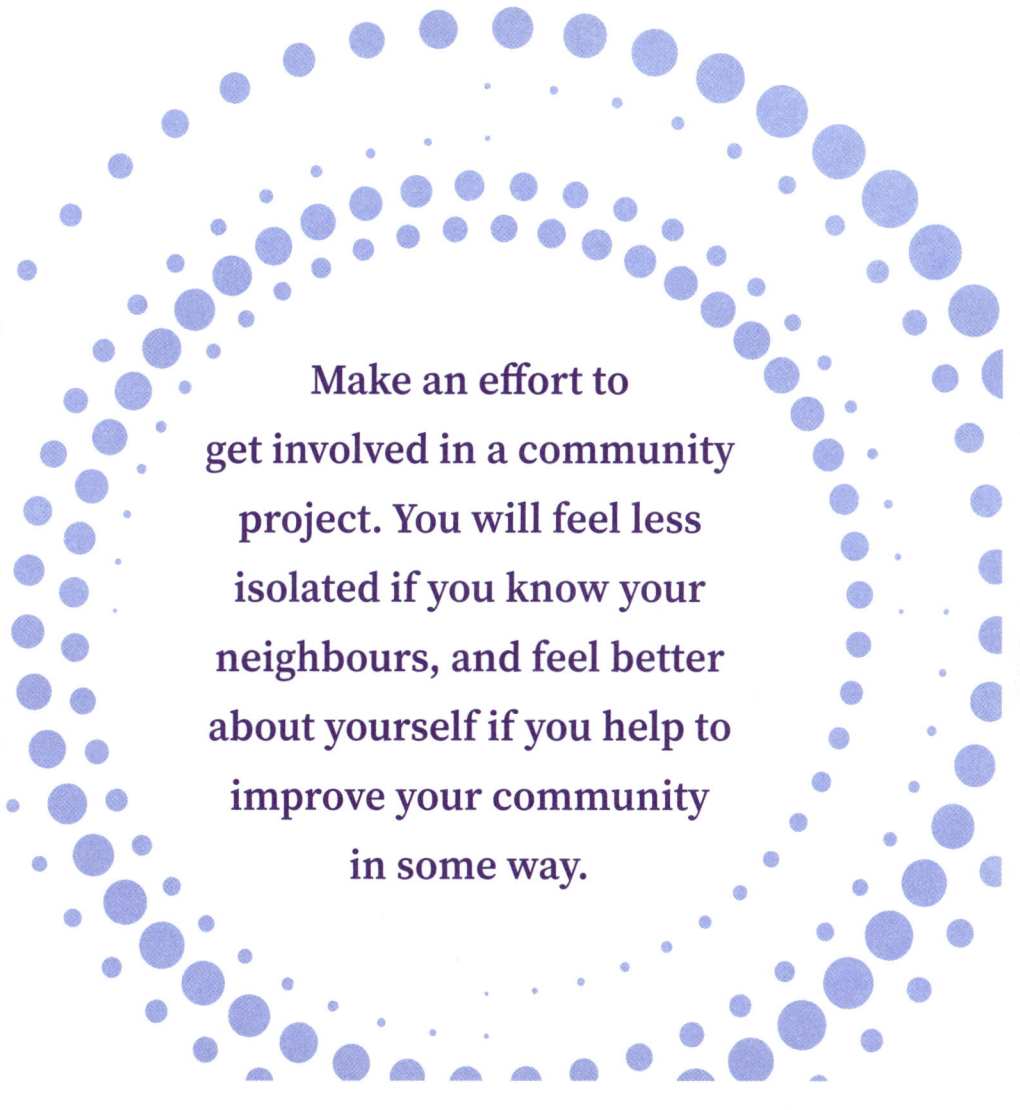

Make an effort to
get involved in a community
project. You will feel less
isolated if you know your
neighbours, and feel better
about yourself if you help to
improve your community
in some way.

It may be necessary temporarily to accept a lesser evil, but one must never label a necessary evil as good.
*Margaret Mead*

Great ideas can grow from the tiniest thought, as long as you carefully nurture that thought with optimism and confidence.

All power ultimately comes from the same place: your own mind.

What you choose not to do is as important as what you choose to do. Refusing to partake in unjust activities is one simple way we can all empower ourselves.

Never feel as though other people are too far above you, too far below you, or too different from you to approach. Introduce yourself, and you will find that the differences between you and them are minor when compared to the similarities.

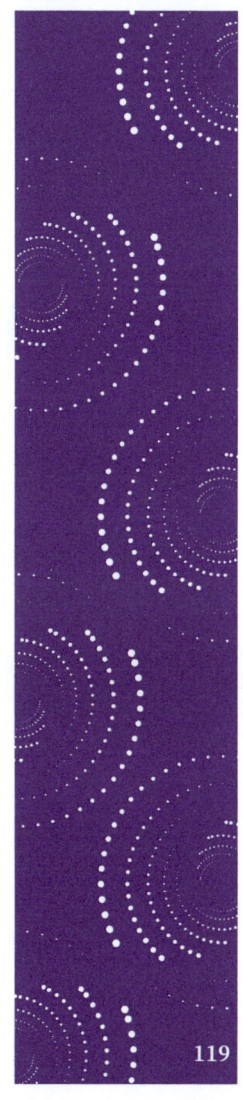

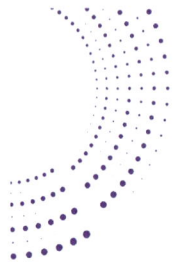

You don't need permission from anyone in order to be happy, but you do need permission from yourself.

**There is no such thing as a completely powerful or completely weak person. We are all a combination of both.**

We are not afraid to look under the bed, or to wash the sheets; we know that life is messy. We know that somebody has to clean it up, and that only if it is cleaned up can we hope to start over, and get better.

*Marsha Norman*

We can all agree
that beauty is in the
eye of the beholder:
what the world needs
is not more beauty
but more
tolerant beholders.

When you feel anxious, count backwards from ten. Take deep breaths. Imagine your worries fading as you count. Repeat these steps until your worries seem manageable again.

The most stable and powerful energy is that which is born from patience.

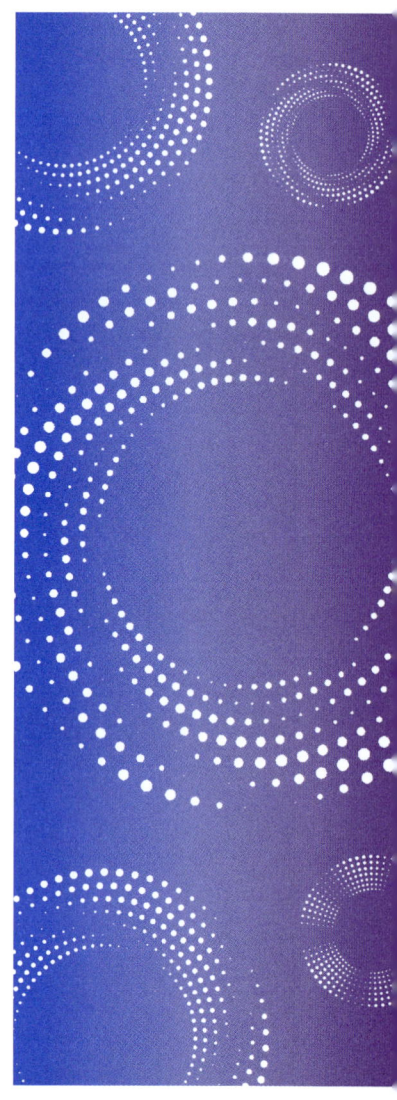

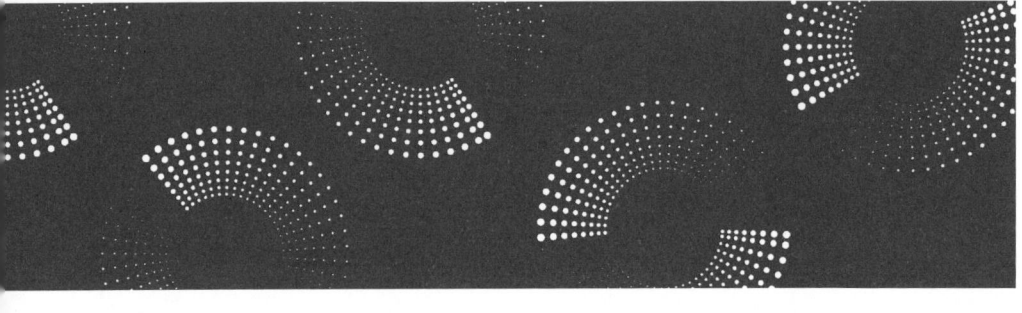

If you take everything
one step at a time,
then nothing will ever
seem very far away.

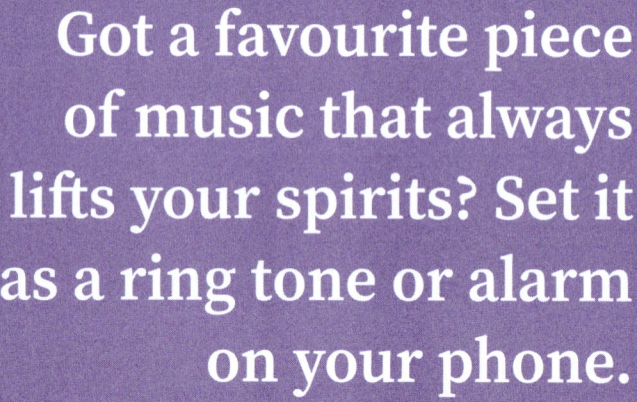

**Got a favourite piece of music that always lifts your spirits? Set it as a ring tone or alarm on your phone.**

When you do nothing, you feel overwhelmed and powerless. But when you get involved, you feel the sense of hope and accomplishment that comes from knowing you are working to make things better.
*Pauline R. Kezer*

Stress steals your energy.
Make sure you have at least
one relaxing activity scheduled
for each and every day.

To be truly unique
you must strive to
stand out, not fit in.

The universe is full of magical
things, patiently waiting for
our wits to grow sharper.
*Eden Phillpotts*

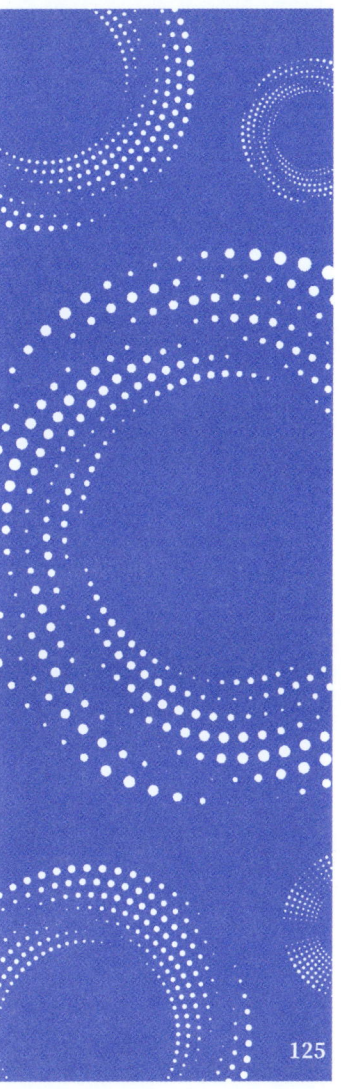

# The grass isn't greener on the other side – it is greener where you water it.

Stand up straight, with your chest out and your head held high. When you have a confident posture, you immediately feel more confident on the inside too.

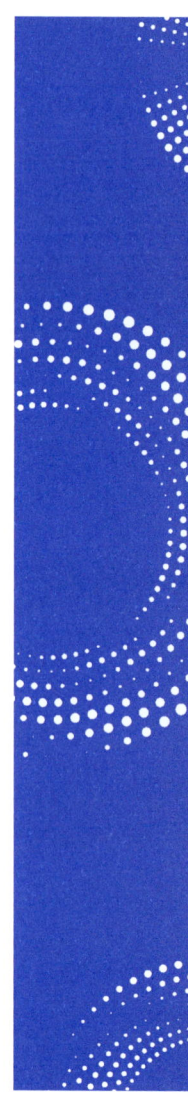

Make today your favourite day of the year. Do the same tomorrow.

Act in order to please yourself, rather than to impress others.

Imagine yourself as full of light, which shines out into the world whenever you smile.

Find a source of positive information. The mainstream news can be relentlessly bleak, so it really helps to supplement it with positive news from a field that you're interested in.

Conditions are never perfect. 'Some day' is a disease that will take your dreams to the grave with you. If it's important to you and you want to do it 'eventually', just do it and correct course along the way.

*Tim Ferriss*

# The Relieved Heart

How can we use empowerment to relieve anxiety around our relationships and to attract new friends and partners?

True confidence is trusting someone else enough to show them your vulnerability.

Try not to look to others for reassurance and validation: only you can really know whether your heart is true, and empowerment means learning to trust your judgement of yourself.

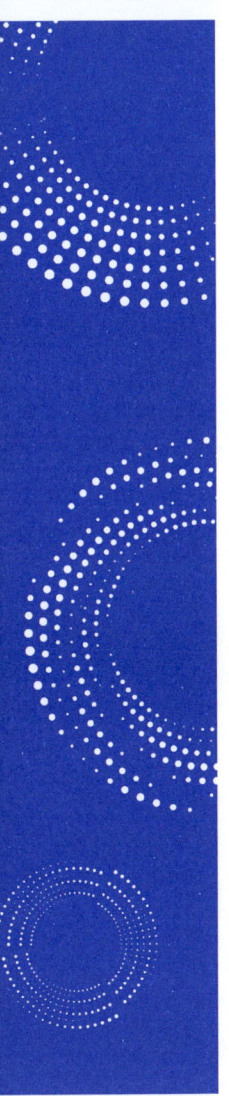

No relationship can survive for long without honesty. Little white lies may be okay from time to time, but always tell the truth about the things that matter.

Don't expect either you or your partner to be perfect. A perfect relationship is not one without any faults, it is one that has grown deep enough to make the faults insignificant.

Nobody enjoys confrontation,
but all successful relationships are
based on good communication.
If something is on your mind,
let others know: don't seethe
quietly or the problem
will only grow worse.

It's easy to point out
the faults of others, but
remember to point out the
strengths of others too.

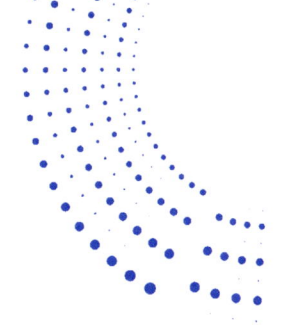

**Learn to tell the difference
between constructive criticism
and destructive criticism.
Only ever give the former, and
value it when it is given to you.**

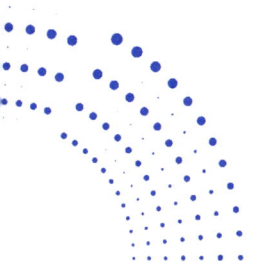

We are more interested in making
others believe we are happy than in
trying to be happy ourselves.
*François de La Rochefoucauld*

I love the man that can smile in trouble, that can gather strength from distress, and grow brave by reflection. 'Tis the business of little minds to shrink, but he whose heart is firm, and whose conscience approves his conduct, will pursue his principles unto death.
*Thomas Paine*

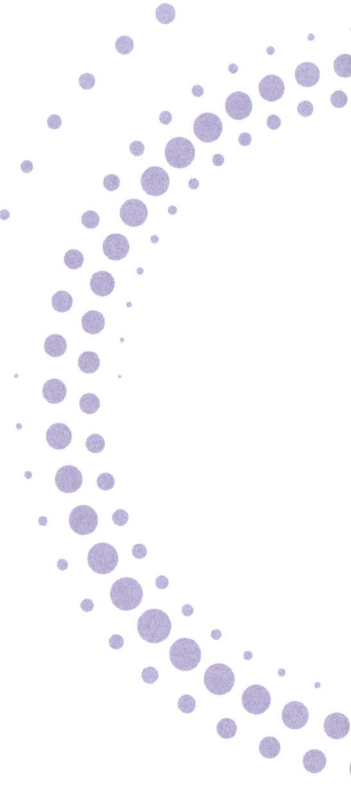

Agree who is going to do the chores, and when. Don't get into arguments about things that don't really matter.

When you become angry, take a couple of seconds to think about your response. Much of the time we don't really mean the first thing that we say in such circumstances.

List the things you argue about with your loved ones, and agree rules that will prevent conflicts arising in the future.

135

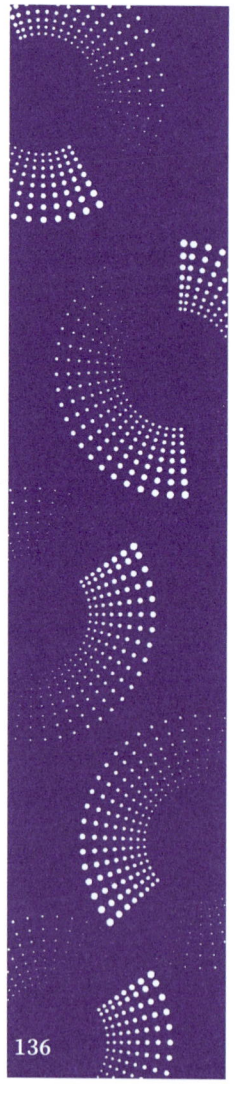

All relationships are works in progress: the moment you stop working at them they begin to fall apart.

To fear love is to fear life, and those who fear life are already three parts dead.

*Bertrand Russell*

Found a new significant other?
Don't abandon your friends in your
excitement; they are the people who
will be there for you should anything
go wrong.

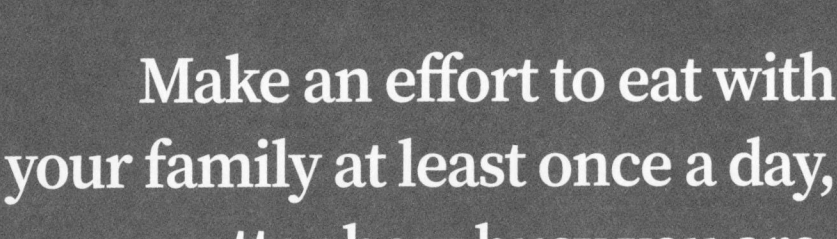

**Make an effort to eat with
your family at least once a day,
no matter how busy you are.**

When you forgive, you heal your own anger and hurt and are able to let love lead again. It's like spring cleaning for your heart.
*Marci Shimoff*

All close families share one common attribute: tolerance.

He who controls others may be powerful, but he who has mastered himself is mightier still.
*Lao Tzu*

Don't abandon friends who have let you down. Place them in a different compartment of your life and wait to see if they can earn your trust again – they might surprise you at some point in the future.

Value those who tell you the truth over those who tell you what you want to hear.

You often have to forgive and forget in order to keep a relationship from failing – and forgetting is often the hardest part.

In a healthy relationship two people are interconnected but never co-dependent.

**Those you love light your way, and in return you must light theirs.**

What a lovely surprise to finally discover how unlonely being alone can be.

*Ellen Burstyn*

Your true wealth is your friends and family, so look after both as if you were guarding treasure.

Although true friendships endure even when contact is limited, you should make a conscious effort to drop a note, email or text to your close friends as often as possible – it reminds them you care about how life is going for them.

You have to become a friend
to someone in order to have
a friend yourself.

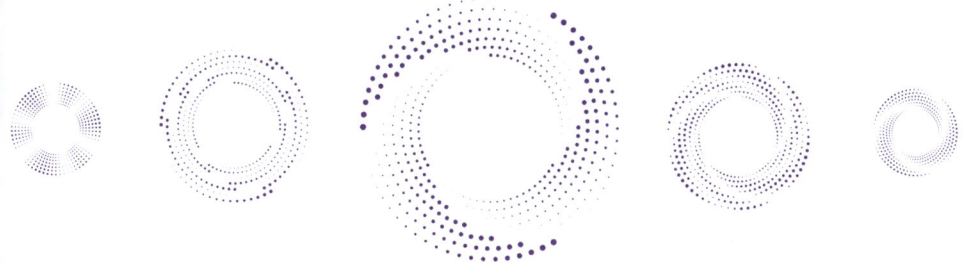

**Empty pockets never held
anyone back. Only empty heads
and empty hearts can do that.**
*Norman Vincent Peale*

# When it comes to friends, quality is far more important than quantity.

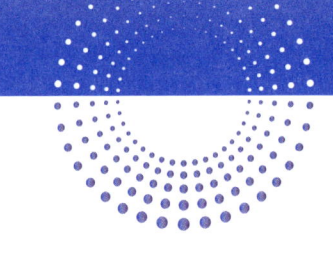

Happiness is a butterfly which, when pursued, is just beyond your grasp ... but, if you will sit down quietly, may alight upon you.

*Nathaniel Hawthorne*

If a loved one has done something to upset you, wait until you are feeling calm, then explain to them what they have done. Don't try to have the conversation while you're hurt or angry.

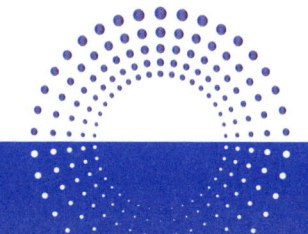

Giving the gift of your friendship is what allows strangers to fulfil their potential and become your friends.

You will never earn the respect of others if you act in ways that cause you to lose respect for yourself.

We can do no great things, only small things with great love.

*Mother Teresa*

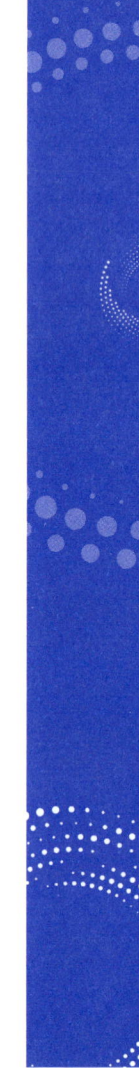

Those who bear grudges eventually fall to their knees under the weight of them.

**The best way to defeat your enemies is to turn them into your friends.**

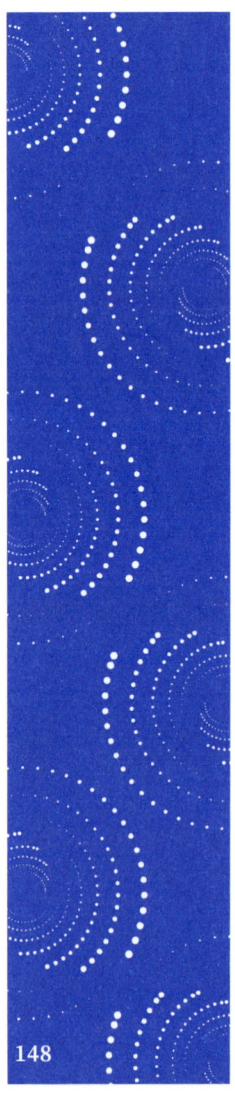

Happiness for a reason is a form of misery because the reason can be taken away from you at any time. To be happy for no reason is the happiness you want to experience. *Vedanta*

Nothing is more empowering than a true and trusted friend.

Why is it that we all tend to judge ourselves by our intentions, but judge others by their actions?

**You show you care about your loved ones when you are too busy, yet still find the time.**

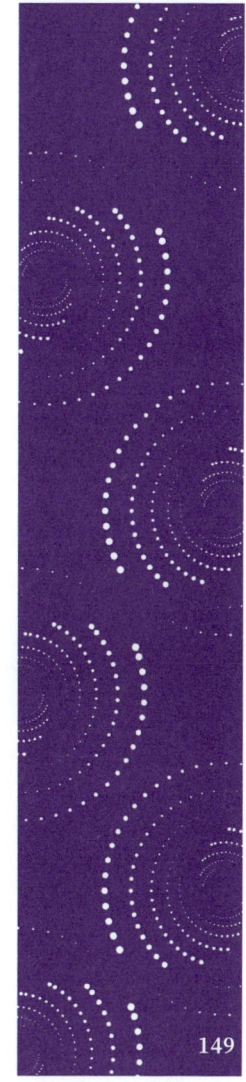

# True love is a partnership, not a competition.

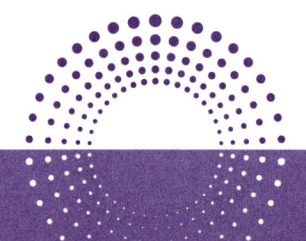

You can't stay in your corner
of the forest waiting for others
to come to you. You have to
go to them sometimes.
*A.A. Milne*

When you don't have to fill the silences you know you're with someone you really feel comfortable being around.

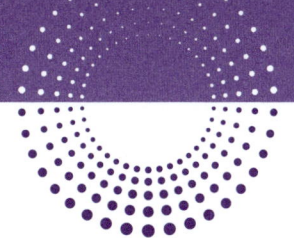

Sometimes when you make a new friend, it is as though you've known them for years. Embrace this feeling rather than trying to analyze it – sometimes the heart just understands things better than the brain.

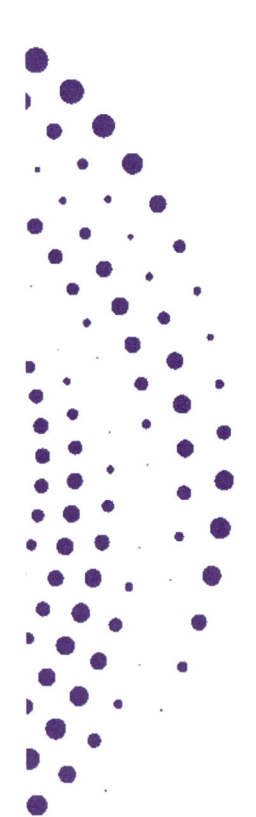

Happiness is like a kiss. You must share it to enjoy it. *Bernard Meltzer*

One of the best ways to catch up with an old friend is to cook them a meal.

People can only be themselves, and you must accept them for who they are. If you spend your time wishing that somebody is more like somebody else, you will always be disappointed.

Live and see,
move around and see more.
*Arab proverb*

**Happiness consists not in having lots of possessions, but in being content with having a few good friends.**

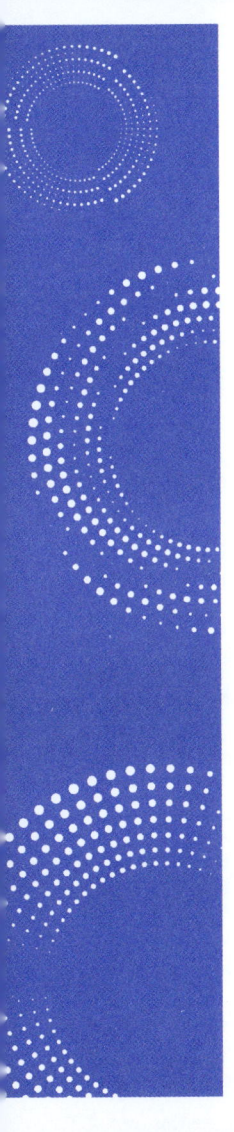

# Harmony in relationships occurs when both parties feel equally valued.

But when you personalize your life, when you make your life a place where you can be yourself, when you do things the way you want to do them, your life feels like your home. And that is a tremendous source of emotional energy.
*Mira Kirshenbaum*

# Never pass on to others what somebody you care about has told you in confidence.

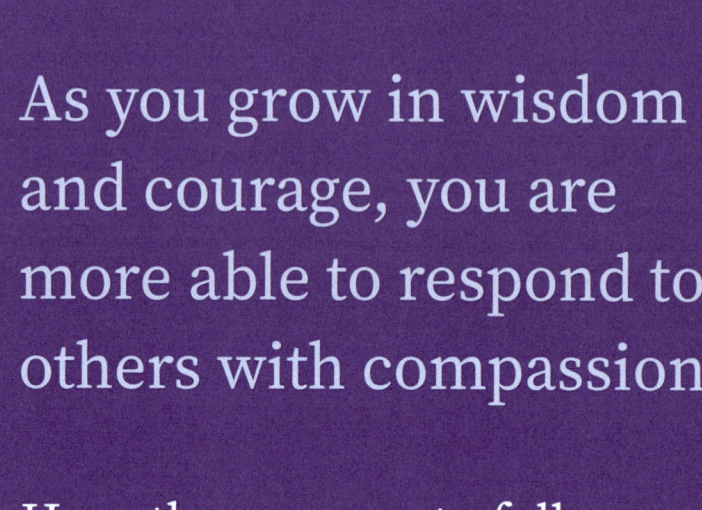

As you grow in wisdom and courage, you are more able to respond to others with compassion.

Have the courage to follow your heart and intuition, they somehow already know what you truly want to become. Everything else is secondary.
*Steve Jobs*

Meeting colleagues after work can sometimes be a revealing experience which shows you a totally different side to someone. Don't judge your workmates solely on how they behave when their guard is up.

What is the point of having anything if you do not have somebody else to share it with?

**Shared interests make relationships easier, but often our relationships with those who have different tastes are the ones that are the most fun.**

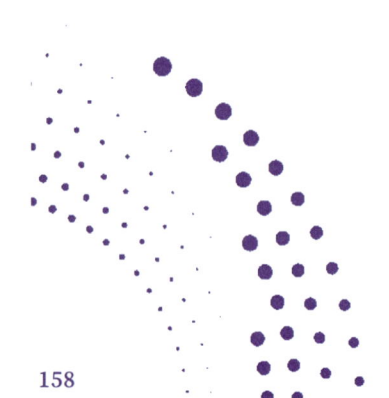

Everyone needs space sometimes. Make sure you find yours when you need it, and always let others find theirs too.

Once in a while,
take the initiative in
your relationships and
suggest an itinerary for a
day rather than asking
others what they'd
like to do.

# Love isn't always easy, but hate is always hard.

Think of your favourite memories, and notice how many of them involve other people being a part of the experience.

**The more anger towards the past you carry in your heart, the less capable you are of loving in the present.**

*Barbara De Angelis*

# When you are kind to others you are also kind to yourself.

**Great people know how to take care of their people. For a great person does not become great by themselves.**
*John Maeda*

Adapt to others, rather than expecting them to adapt to you.

Treat everybody as your equal – and remember this applies to those in high-status positions as well as those in low-status ones.

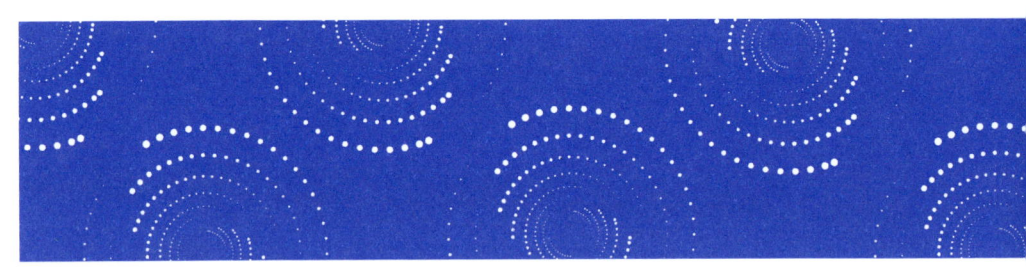

We are not held back by the love we didn't receive in the past, but by the love we're not extending in the present.

*Marianne Williamson*

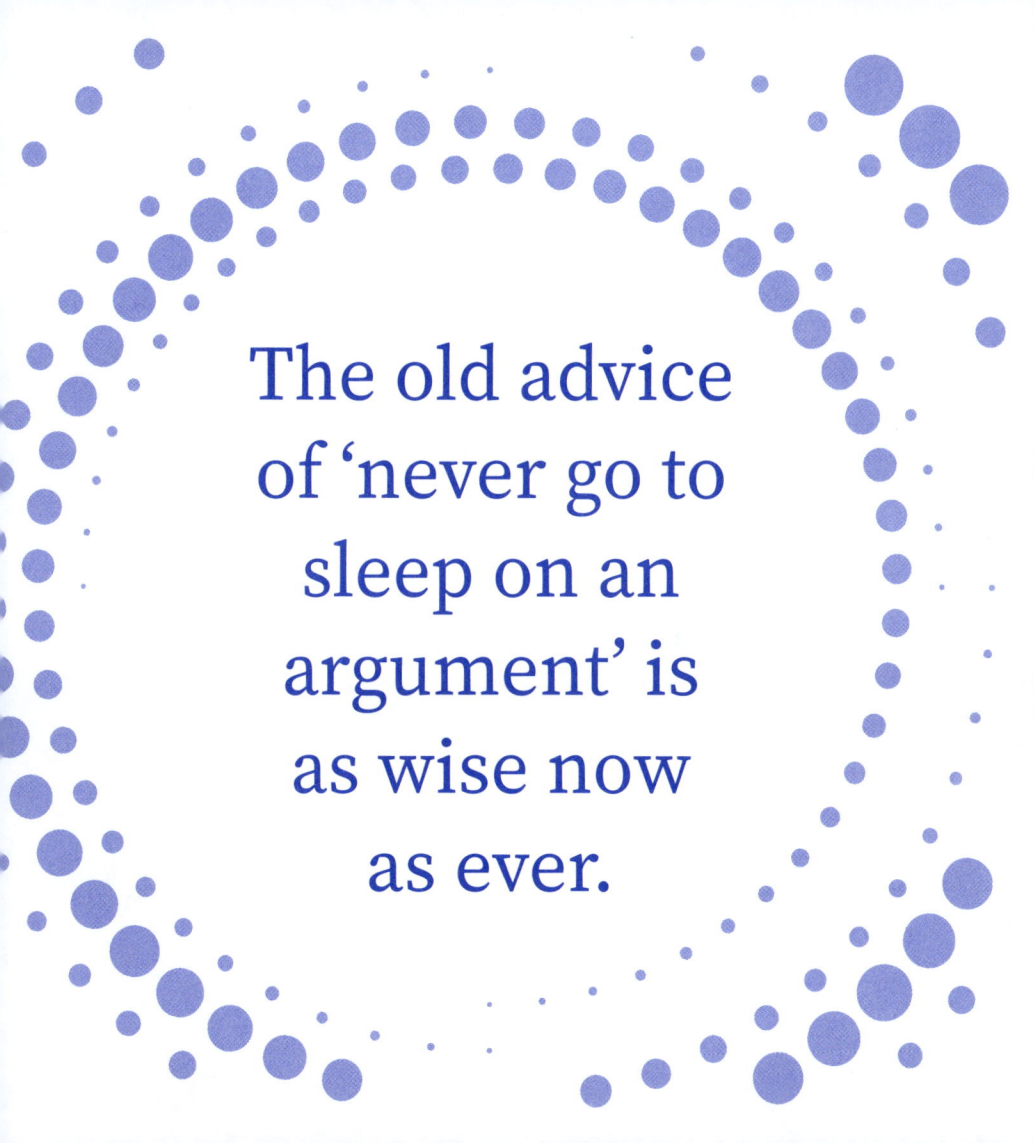

The old advice
of 'never go to
sleep on an
argument' is
as wise now
as ever.

Don't confuse the carelessness or stupidity of others with malice.

We come to resemble the people we surround ourselves with – so choose your friends wisely!

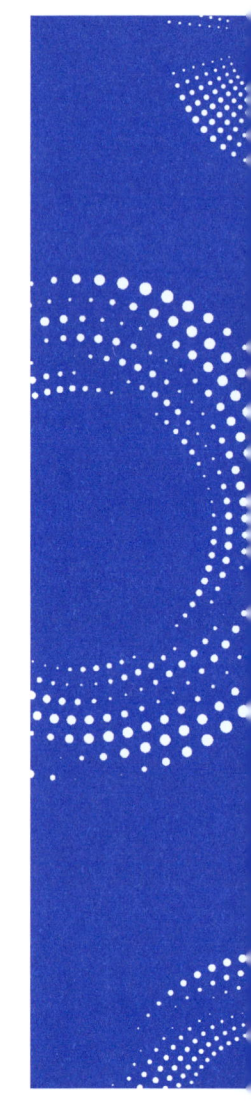

**If you find qualities you admire in others, cultivate them in yourself.**

Wealth is the ability to fully experience life.
*Henry David Thoreau*

Remember that the truest friend any of us has is ourselves.

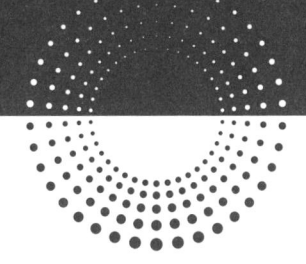

Throw your dreams into space like a kite, and you do not know what it will bring back: a new life, a new friend, a new love, a new country.

*Anaïs Nin*

You can never have too many friends. Don't allow certain relationships to wither just because others are easier to maintain.

**Friendships, like fine wines, improve with age.**

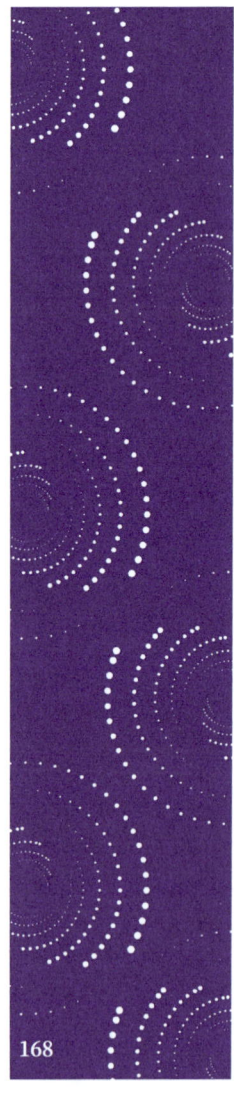

# Don't just chat with your loved ones – ask their advice on important matters and, above all, listen to that advice.

Even through the toughest times, friends share smiles and laughter. If you have a friend who only seems to share misery then you need to reassess that relationship.

All blame is a waste of time.
No matter how much fault you
find with another, and regardless
of how much you blame him,
it will not change you.
*Wayne Dyer*

**In the end, the way
you behave towards
others defines who
you actually are.**

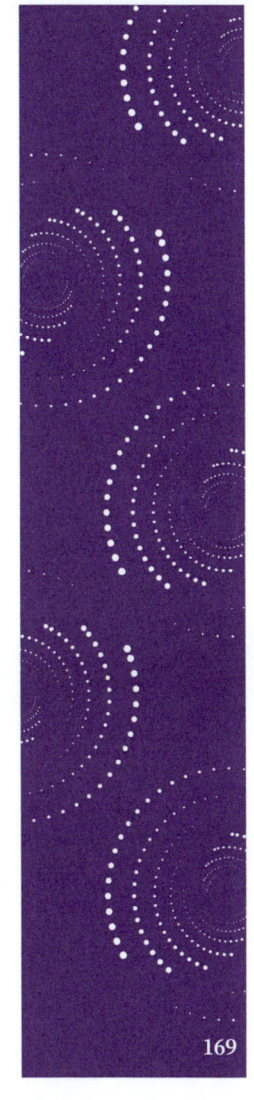

# Never try to change anybody who does not want to change.

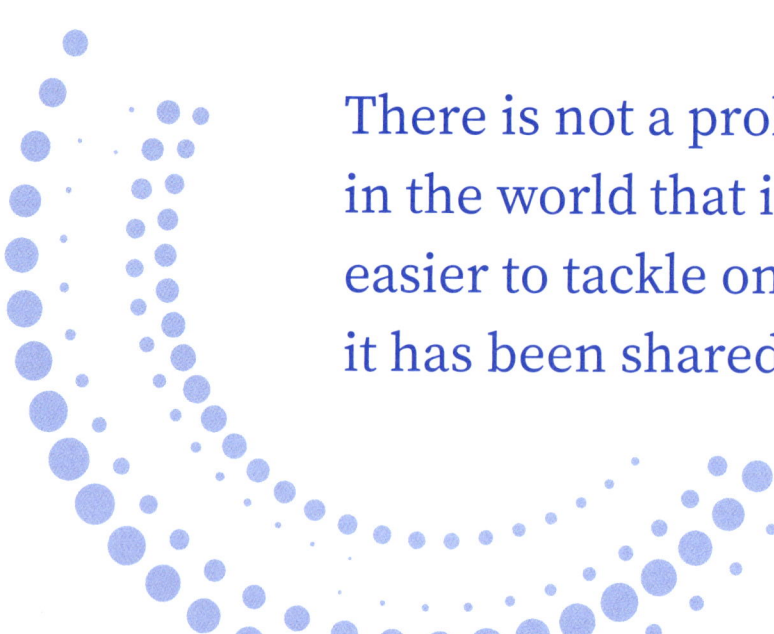

There is not a problem in the world that is not easier to tackle once it has been shared.

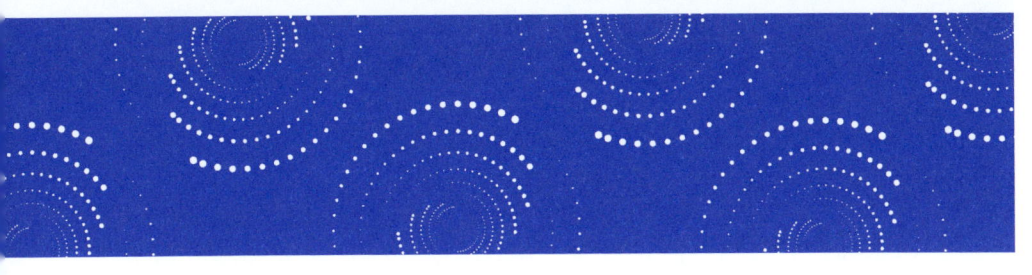

Live your life from your heart.
Share from your heart. And your story
will touch and heal people's souls.
*Melody Beattie*

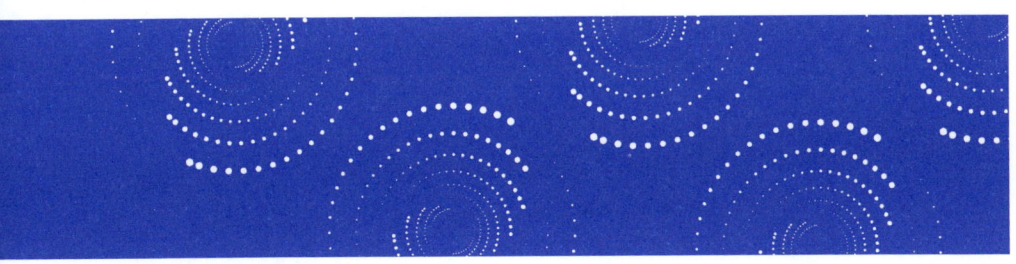

No person is ever too old,
too young, too rich or too
poor to become a friend.

Remember to praise what children do right, rather than just scolding them for the things they do wrong; approval will build their confidence for adult life.

---

**Very few people are really lazy, they just don't have goals that inspire them. Remember to follow your heart: what inspires you?**

---

To befriend an elderly person is to have a fount of wisdom at your side.

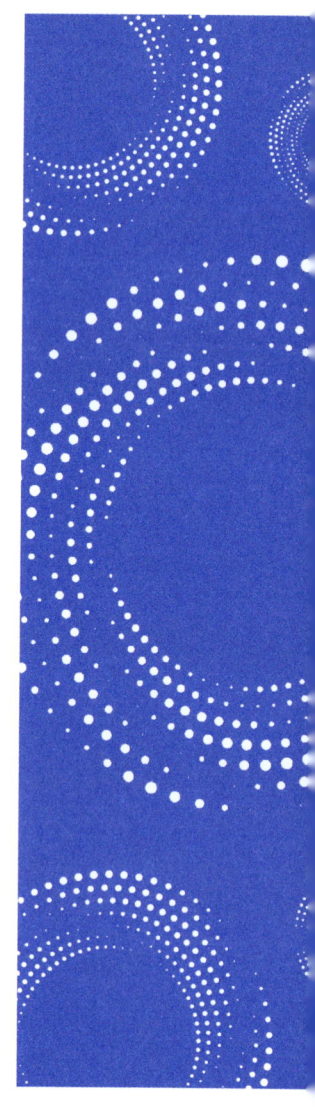

As I go through all kinds of feelings and experiences in my journey through life – delight, surprise, chagrin, dismay – I hold this question as a guiding light: 'What do I really need right now to be happy?' What I come to over and over again is that only qualities as vast and deep as love, connection and kindness will really make me happy in any sort of enduring way.

*Sharon Salzberg*

Nothing you experience in life has not been experienced by someone else before. Friendship is all about sharing experiences and exchanging advice.

**If there must be trouble, let it be in my day, that my child may have peace.**

*Thomas Paine*

# You don't really ever make friends – your friends make you.

Friends on social network sites are all well and good, but don't confuse them with real-world friends. There's still no substitute for a friend you can share a hug with.

It is far easier to be angry than it is to be patient, but patience brings a controlled response and anger often leads to us losing control.

Life is not measured by the number of breaths we take, but by the moments that take our breath away.
*Maya Angelou*

When your loved ones are lost, make sure they know the way to reach your door.

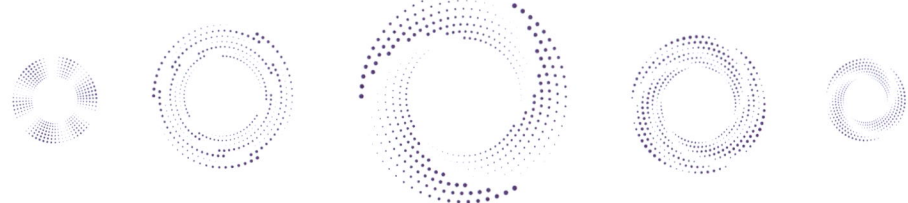

There is no more empowering act than fixing a friendship that was previously broken.

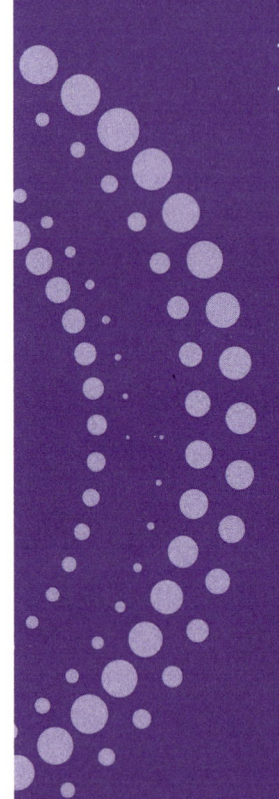

Don't underestimate the joy and companionship that animals can bring.

Your life feels different on you, once you greet death and understand your heart's position. You wear your life like a garment from the mission bundle sale ever after – lightly because you realize you paid nothing for it, cherishing because you know you won't ever come by such a bargain again.

*Louise Erdrich*

To be happy alone
is to befriend
yourself.

Love is life's end, but never ending.
Love is life's wealth, never spent,
but ever spending. Love is life's reward,
rewarded in rewarding.
*Herbert Spencer*

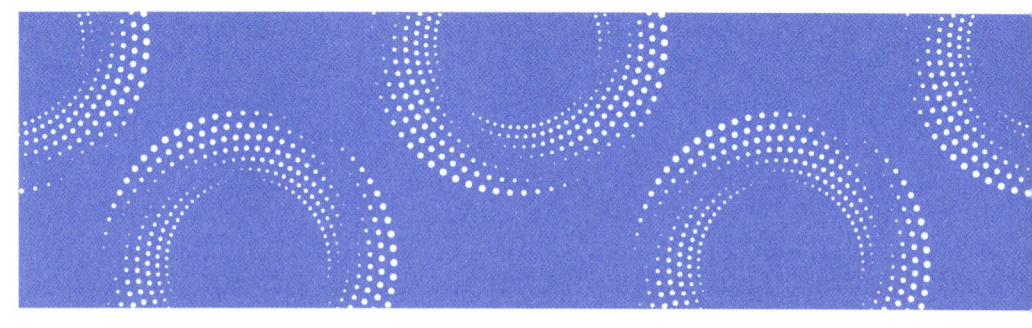

Nobody who has lots of interests is short of friends: one of the easiest ways to meet new people is to take up a new hobby.

**You can get everything in life you want if you will just help enough other people get what they want.**

*Zig Ziglar*

What do you really know about your friends? Many of us know surprisingly little when we stop and think about it. Make the effort to find out more, if your friends are happy to share the information.

**You don't have to travel to the ends of the earth in order to find love – but you do have to travel beyond your own front door.**

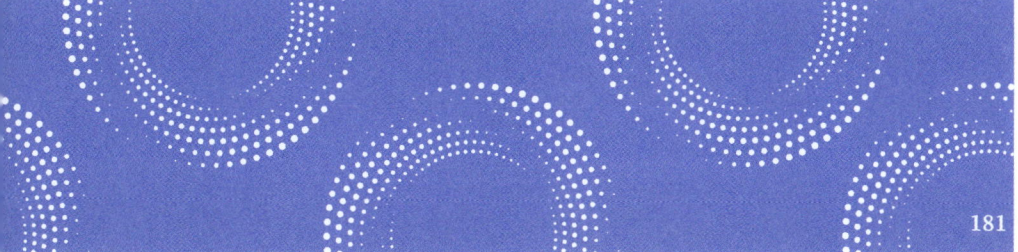

It is amazing how much stress can be lifted from your shoulders just by sharing a glass of wine and a laugh with a loved one.

We can only be said to be alive in those moments when our hearts are conscious of our treasures.

*Thornton Wilder*

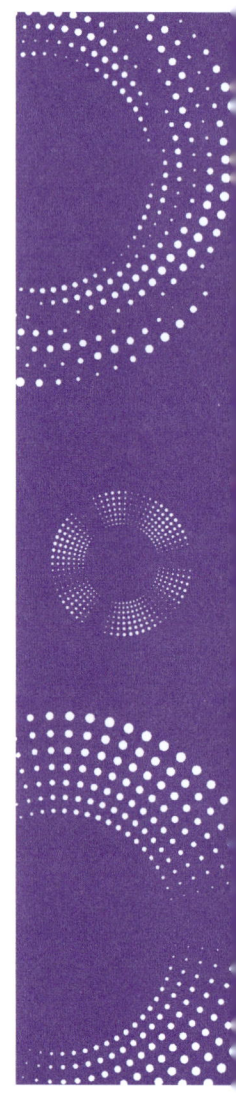

# Strive to make all of your friends your best friends.

There are rare occasions when you do have to walk away from somebody that you previously thought of as a friend. Don't stay friends with somebody simply because you are afraid of change: if you are in a hurtful or toxic relationship, then it is not really a friendship.

We don't get to choose the partners and friends of our friends: make an effort to respect the choices of your friends, though, even if you feel they may be choosing unwisely.

Even if you search the entire world you will not find anybody who is more deserving of your love and affection than you are yourself.

**In action a great heart is the chief qualification. In work, a great head.**
*Arthur Schopenhauer*

**Relationships require continual effort, just as we require food and water.**

Life is sometimes a struggle but – thankfully – we are all in it together.

**Think where man's glory most begins and ends, And say my glory was I had such friends.**

*W. B. Yeats*

Don't get on with your in-laws? Remember that they are responsible for bringing into the world the person you love.

**Thanks to social networking sites, it has never been easier to find lost friends and acquaintances. Finding an old friend is often even more rewarding than making a new friend.**

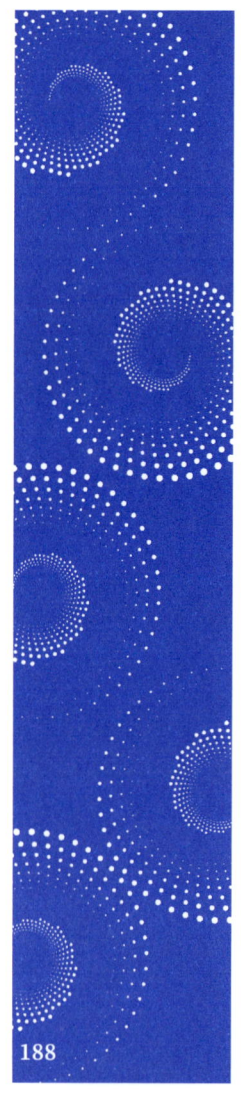

Love is not an affectionate feeling, but a steady wish for the loved person's ultimate good as far as it can be obtained.
*C.S. Lewis*

Sometimes it feels as though we give more than we receive. In any meaningful relationship the books balance eventually – but often we don't realize it until we view the relationship over the course of an entire lifetime.

Think of an especially wonderful memory that you shared with a loved one. Surprise them by celebrating the anniversary of that event.

It is the shared struggles, not just the shared laughs, that make relationships meaningful.

# Love takes up where rational thought leaves off.

Forget about the fast lane. If you want to fly, just harness your power to your passion. Honor your calling. Everybody has one. Trust your heart and success will come to you.

*Oprah Winfrey*

# You are loved. Remind yourself of this every day.

How lucky I am to have something that makes saying good-bye so hard.

*A.A. Milne*

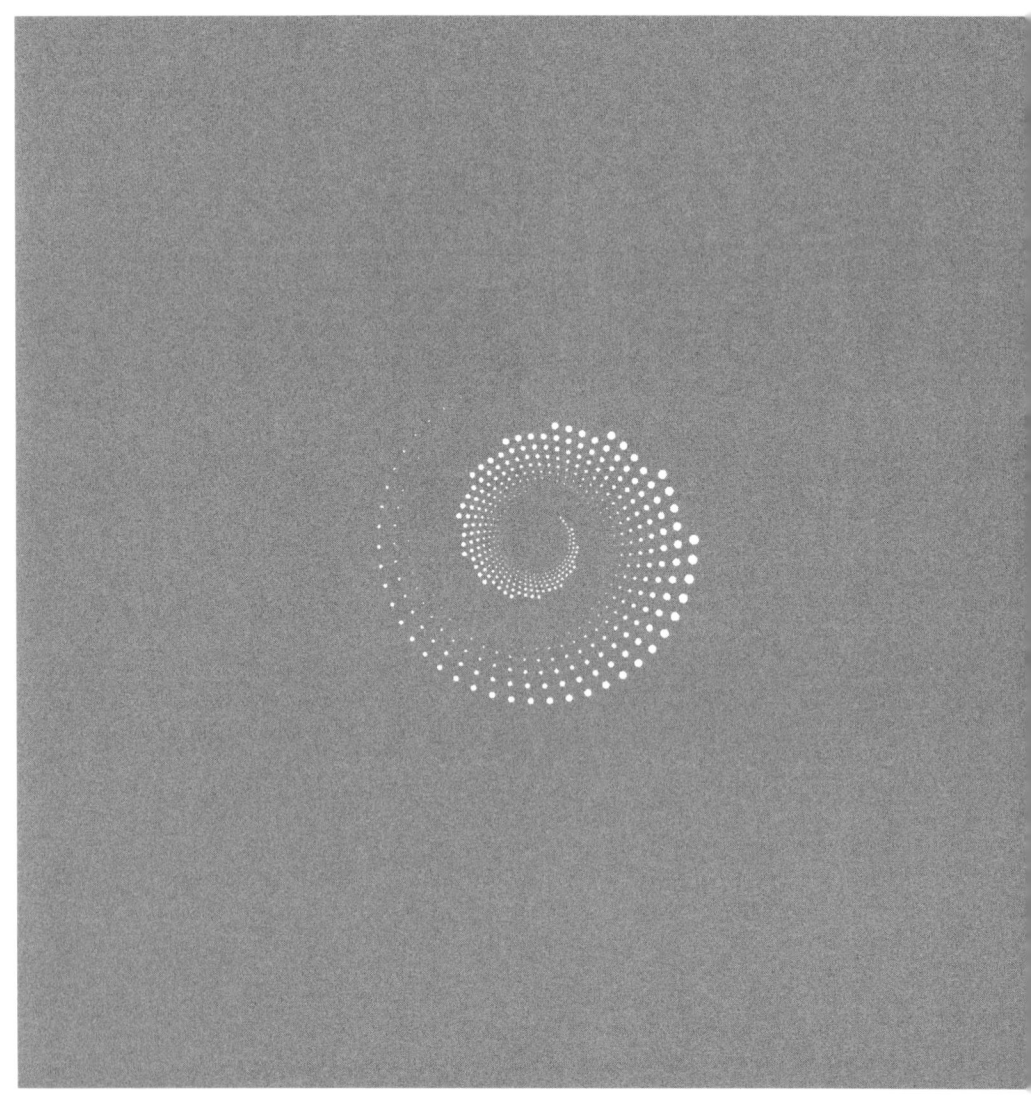

# Stress-free at Work

In this section we explore how empowerment can make us less anxious and more productive in the workplace.

A leader is best when people barely know he exists. When his work is done, his aim fulfilled, they will say: we did it ourselves.

*Lao Tzu*

Big success means taking big risks – which means having big confidence.

# When you feel great, everyone is more responsive to you – it's a virtuous circle.

You don't always get what you deserve in life – but it is the honours that you deserve rather than those you are awarded that will define how successful you yourself feel.

Never continue in
a job you don't enjoy. If you're
happy in what you're doing, you'll
like yourself, you'll have inner
peace. And if you have that, along
with physical health, you will
have had more success than you
could possibly have imagined.
*Johnny Carson*

The more things you do,
the more you can do.
*Lucille Ball*

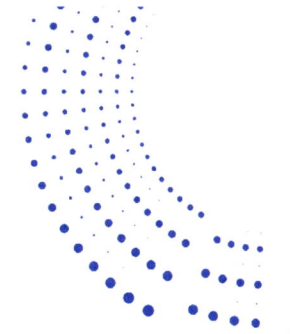

Often the most difficult part
of a task is realizing that there
is a simple way to do it.

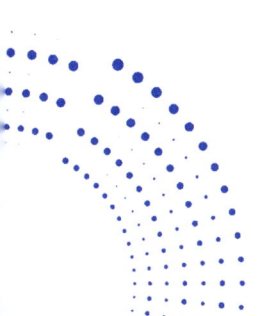

**You lead people most
effectively when you
walk behind them.**

Don't bite off more than you can chew. Lean into the joy of saying 'no' sometimes.

Remember to work wholeheartedly when at work and relax fully when you are done.

**Don't just 'sell and forget'. The customer you build a relationship with will return time and time again.**

Always write out a weekly and then a daily to do list so that you can capture exactly what is important and, vitally, what is not and can be ignored.

Learn when not to take 'no' for an answer. A little persistence can go a long way.

Don't aim for perfection, just aim for improvement – eventually you'll find yourself closer to perfection than you ever thought possible.

Work in bursts, then rest. An hour of truly productive work will leave you feeling temporarily drained, so recharge regularly, even if it is only a five-minute break or a walk to get a drink of water.

Would you hire yourself, if you were looking for staff? If so, what are your strengths? If not, what do you need to brush up on?

Repeat this mantra: you are only human. Be the best you can be, but don't fall into the trap of taking on the impossible.

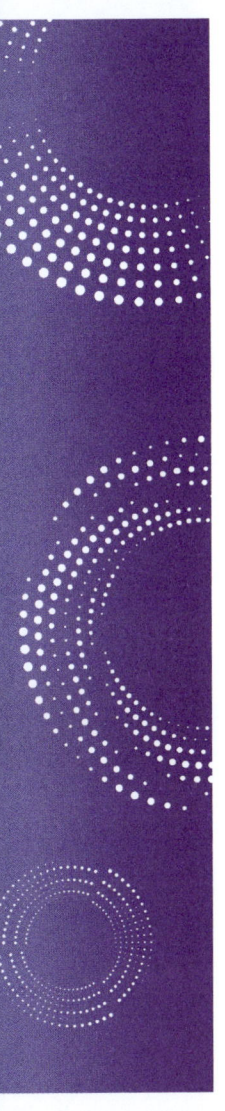

Rely on yourself rather than others and you'll soon be thought of as the most reliable person in your workplace.

I guess we all like to be recognized not for one piece of fireworks, but for the ledger of our daily work.
*Neil Armstrong*

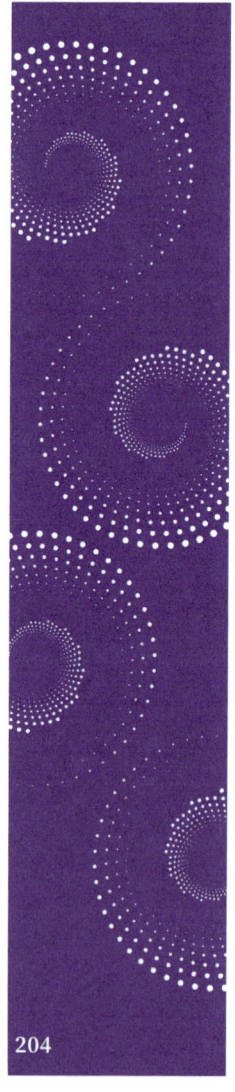

Word of mouth is by far the most effective form of advertising. Concentrate on building a reputation for fairness and efficiency and you'll soon have all the orders you can handle.

The secret of getting ahead
is getting started.
*Sally Berger*

---

**Laughter in the workplace
is good for productivity.**

---

Compete against your own
potential, not against that
of your colleagues.

Don't fall for the spin – neither the spin others tell you, nor the spin you tell yourself.

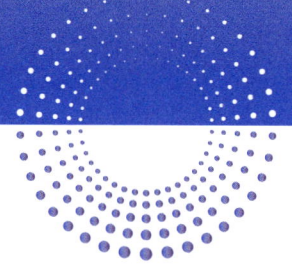

Making money isn't the backbone of our guiding purpose; making money is the by-product of our guiding purpose.

*Warren Buffett*

Give yourself the time and space to dream. Good ideas can transform your work, but they rarely come unless you create the right conditions for them to grow in.

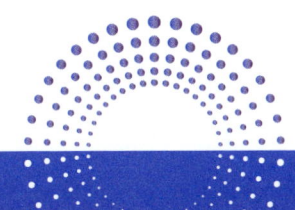

Rather than worrying about the future, roll up your sleeves and begin to create it.

It is far more effective to persuade somebody that doing a job is important than to just force them to do what you want.

Half the battle of life is discovering what you are good at. Once you know this, everything else becomes easier.

Choose a job you love and
you will never have to work
a day in your life.

*Confucius*

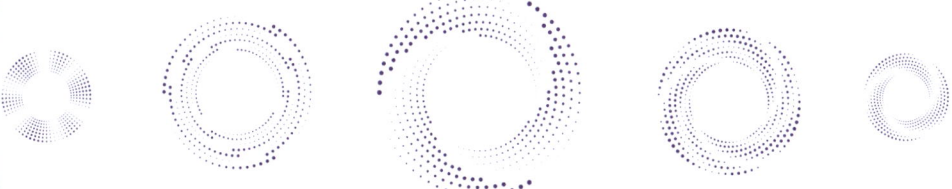

**Wishing you had more takes
up valuable time that could be
spent doing the work needed to
get what you really want.**

**Don't worry about not having all of the necessary skills to get a job done: the most important skill in any line of work is common sense.**

Success is not the key to happiness. Happiness is the key to success. If you love what you are doing, you will be successful.

*Albert Schweitzer*

Don't try to hide your true self while at work in order to make yourself look better. You will become a more valuable asset by being who you really are.

When hard work becomes second nature, it ceases to be hard work.

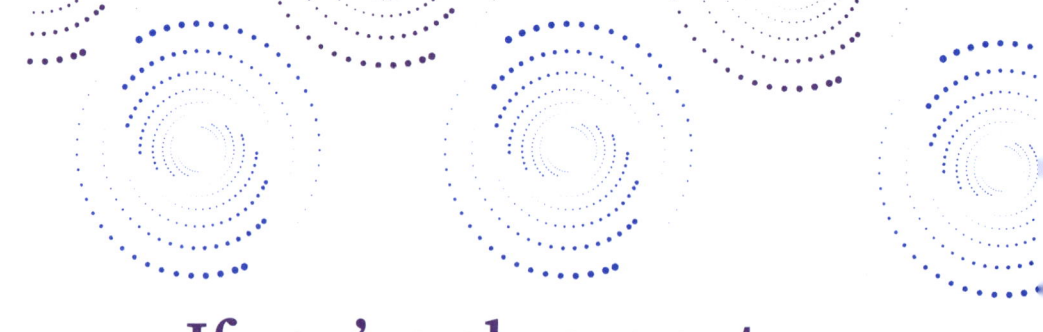

If you've always got your
shoulder to the wheel,
you might well end up
not being able to see where
you are pushing it to.

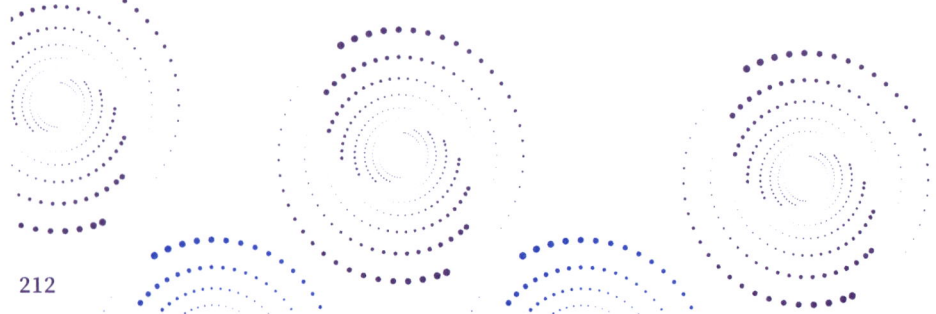

Those who
learn to co-operate
well with others multiply
their power many times over.

---

**Those who say it cannot be
done should not interrupt
the person doing it.**
*Chinese proverb*

# The way to riches is via rich thinking.

No matter what you are selling, in the end you are selling yourself. Make that self valuable to others and you will have no shortage of customers willing to buy.

The biggest opportunities are those that others have overlooked, so don't be afraid to seek them in unusual places.

If you're interested,
you'll do what's convenient;
if you're committed, you'll
do whatever it takes.

*John Assaraf*

Having time off is great, but don't resent the return to work. True happiness doesn't lie in doing nothing, but in being busy doing something worthwhile.

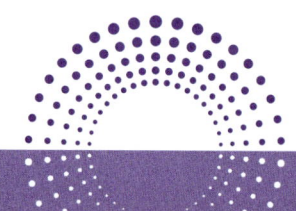

**Formal education will make you a living; self-education will make you a fortune.**

*Jim Rohn*

# Even better than winning a battle is avoiding a battle in the first place.

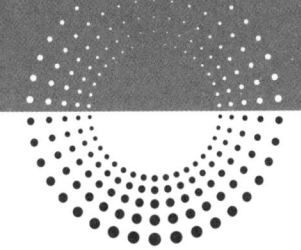

Learn to watch for signs that you are becoming frustrated. When you see those signs, stop for a while and put your problems into perspective. You'll see that you've really been battling against yourself, not against the problem.

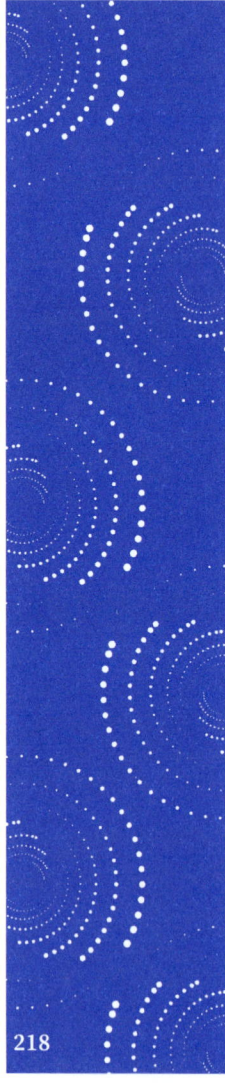

Your work is going to fill a large part of your life, and the only way to be truly satisfied is to do what you believe is great work. And the only way to do great work is to love what you do. If you haven't found it yet, keep looking, and don't settle. As with all matters of the heart, you'll know when you find it. *Steve Jobs*

One of the mistakes we all tend to make is that of trying too hard. It is better in the long run to work methodically than in wild bursts.

Recognizing good advice is a skill that requires practice. Following good advice requires even greater skill.

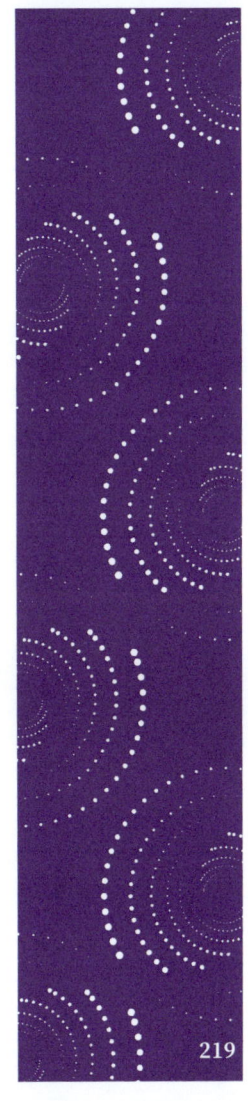

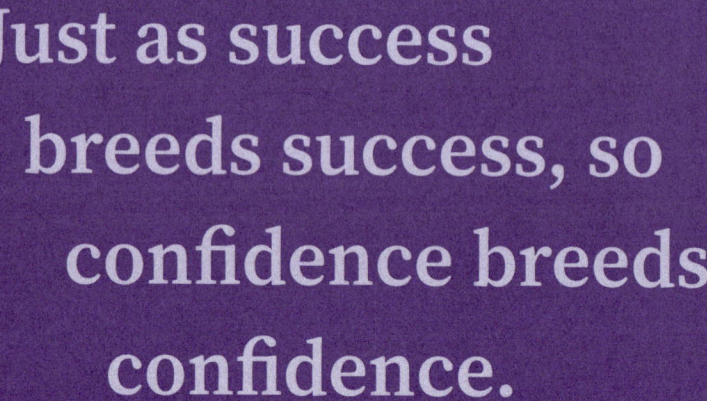

**Just as success breeds success, so confidence breeds confidence.**

If only we could bottle the sense of achievement we get when we've done a good job, we would always feel confident about getting the next job done.

Nobody ever prospered without a prosperous attitude.

Remember that we are all human beings, not human doings – so take the time to *be* and not just *do*.

**The mode in which the inevitable comes to pass is through effort.**
*Oliver Wendell Holmes*

If something is beyond your reach, visualize possessing it, and it will suddenly seem an awful lot closer.

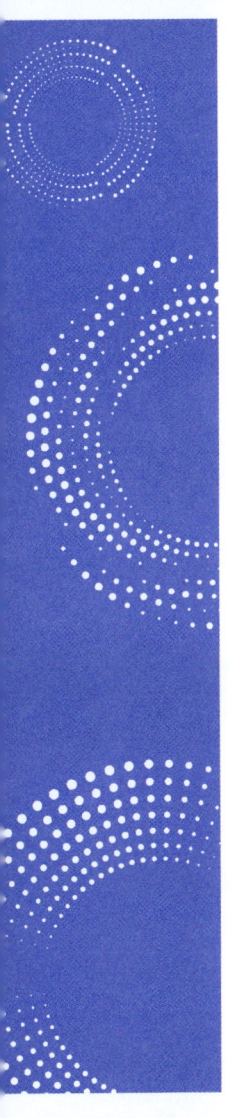

Contemplating the results of a job well done is one of the great treasures of life.

**Throwing yourself into your work can sometimes blow away all the doubts and fears you had about your life.**

Learn to be happy when others succeed, not just when you yourself succeed, and you will be happy much more often.

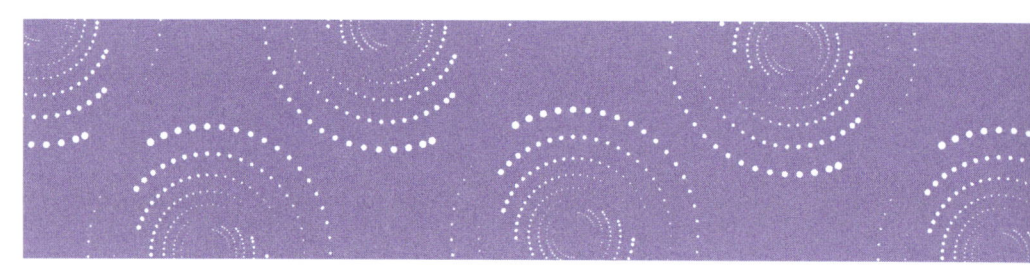

**Truly empowered people only want to be better than themselves, not change other people.**

If a man is called to be a street-sweeper, he should sweep streets even as Michelangelo painted, or Beethoven composed music, or Shakespeare wrote poetry. He should sweep streets so well that all the hosts of heaven and earth will pause to say, here lived a great street-sweeper who did his job well.

*Martin Luther King, Jr.*

# The Spirit of Empowerment

It's one thing to act in a self-assured manner, but another thing to truly feel powerful within. Here we see how empowerment is vital to combatting the feelings of anxiety that can arise.

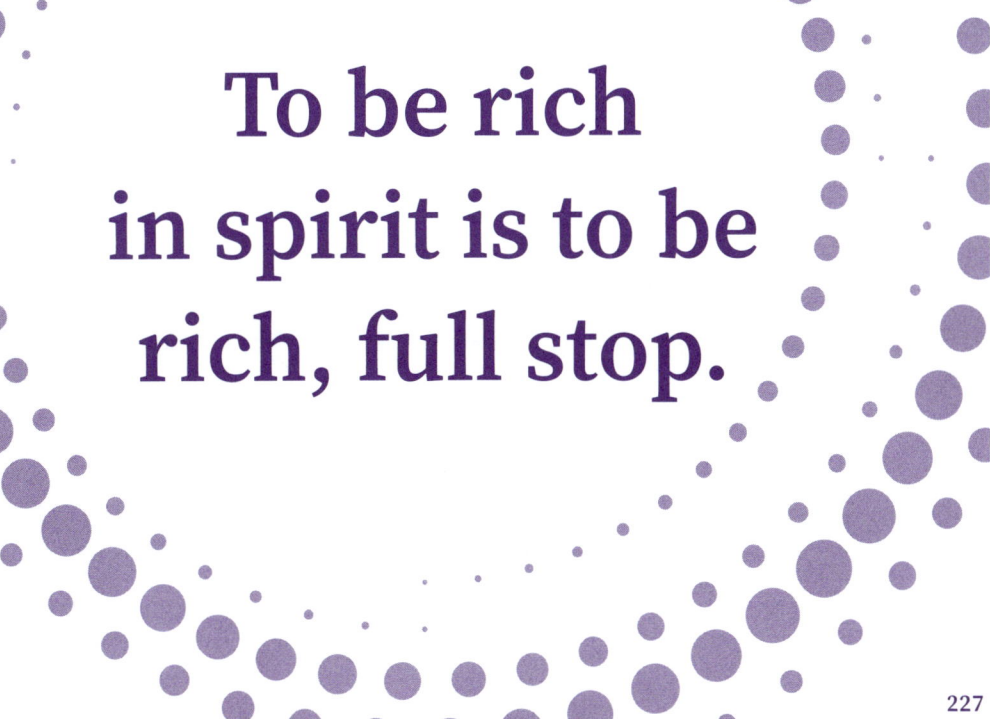

To be rich
in spirit is to be
rich, full stop.

The hardest battle to win in life is the battle we fight against our own negative thoughts.

Life can only be lived in one direction, so embrace change, and live each day without looking back.

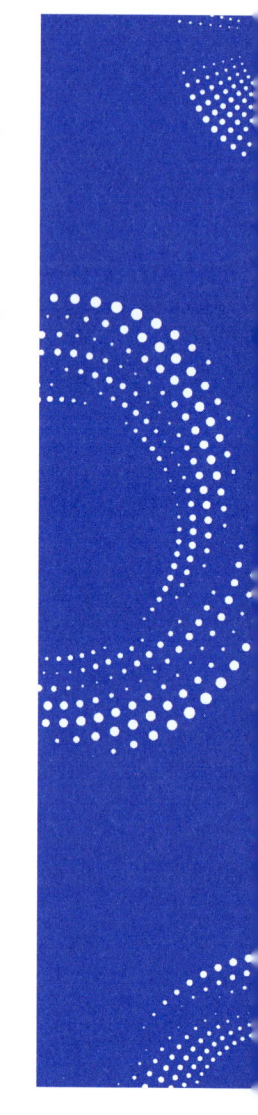

Shoot for the moon.
Even if you miss, you'll
land among the stars.
*Les Brown*

If you never take a
chance then you never
win: the trick is to
always know when the
odds are in your favour.

**Life is worth living only if we ourselves make it worth living.**

The trappings of success are called 'trappings' for a reason.

To dare is to lose one's footing momentarily. To not dare is to lose oneself.
*Søren Kierkegaard*

The softest things in the world overcome the hardest things in the world.
*Lao Tzu*

The only real heaven lies within us, not above us.

Nobody's life is small or insignificant: every life is equally special and meaningful, including yours.

If you want to change the world, you have to start by changing yourself.

# Wonderful actions are far more powerful than wonderful thoughts or words.

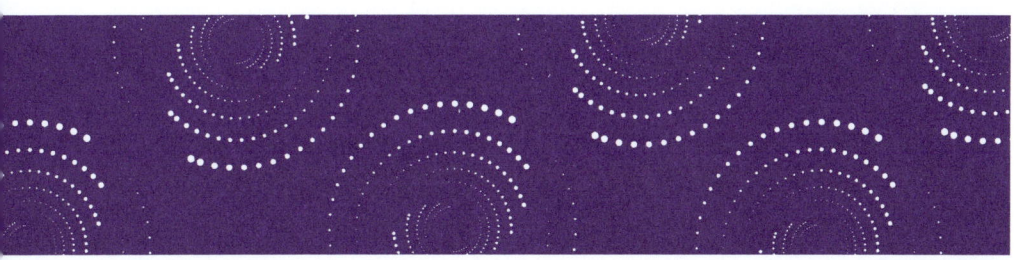

Whether you succeed or not is irrelevant, there is no such thing. Making your unknown known is the important thing.

*Georgia O'Keeffe*

233

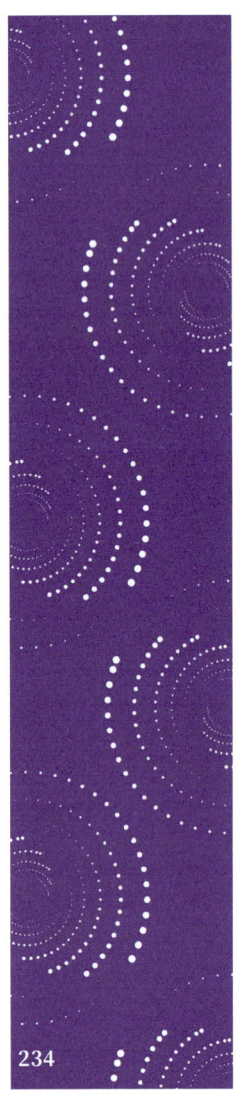

# To get better at anything you first have to want to get better.

Be honest about what causes you anxiety. You can often place the cause at someone else's door when really it is an issue that lies within yourself. Take back your power and you will find relief from anxiety.

**The double truth of feeling totally unimportant and at the same time of uppermost importance is of great help in mastering life in its various aspects.**

*Hans Taeger*

Not even death is strong enough to destroy our good deeds.

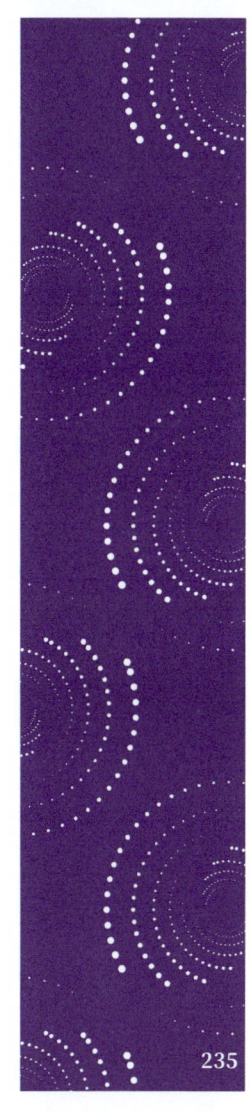

Having convictions does not mean believing you are 100 per cent right and others are 100 per cent wrong. To act in an empowered fashion you need to recognize the countless shades of grey, not believe that life is black and white.

**Those who throw their weight around are usually perceived as weak, rather than strong.**

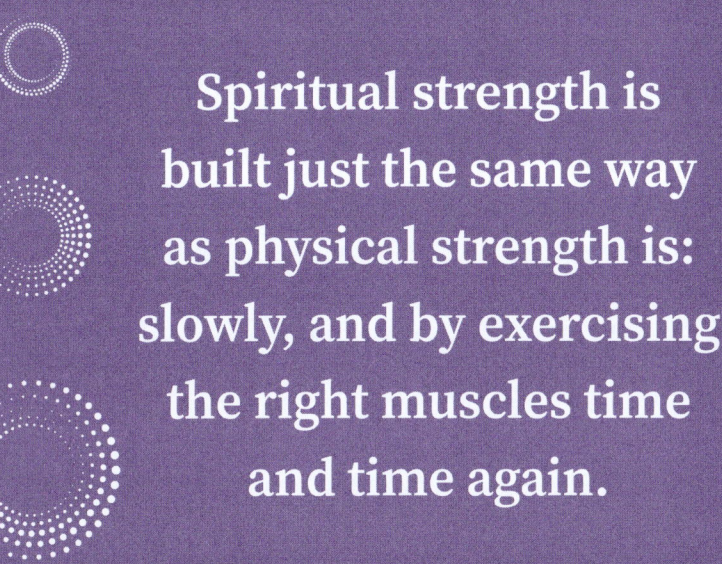

**Spiritual strength is
built just the same way
as physical strength is:
slowly, and by exercising
the right muscles time
and time again.**

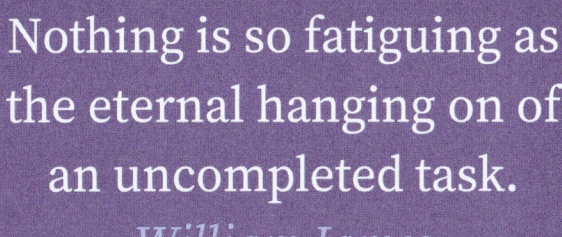

Nothing is so fatiguing as
the eternal hanging on of
an uncompleted task.
*William James*

**Life should be savoured like a fine wine, not gulped down. Take your time and enjoy every mouthful.**

Empowerment is not about always being strong, it is about being strong at the right times. It is as much about timing as it is about strength.

Even when you're alone, you should act as if others can see your every move.

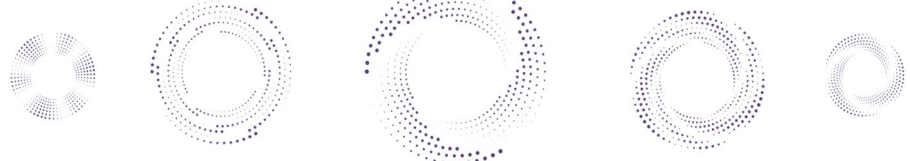

Apologizing does not make you look weak if you believe you are in the wrong. Apologizing when you believe you are in the right, however, is a sure sign you are allowing yourself to be bullied.

The bigger the change that is needed, the more gentle you need to be – with yourself and with others.

We only stop growing physically. We grow spiritually every day, as long as we exercise our inner strength.

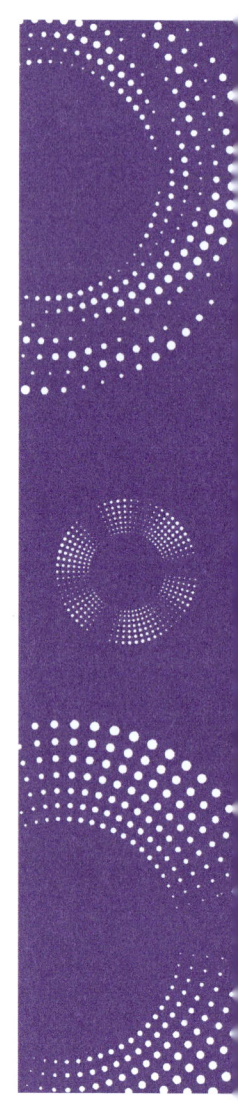

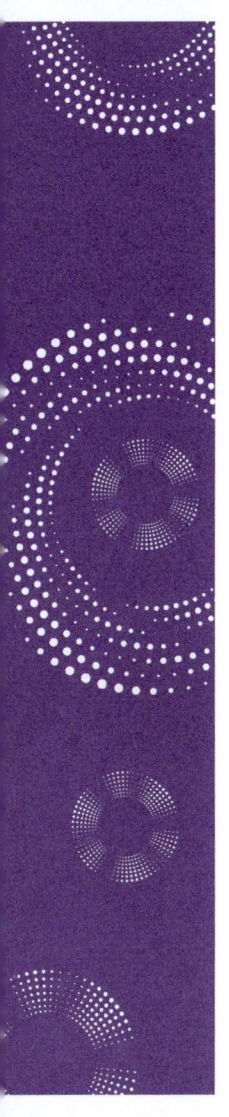

**I always wondered why somebody didn't do something about that. Then I realized I was somebody.**
*Lily Tomlin*

Where do you really want to get to, and what is stopping you? Write these down, and refer to them often. Tackle the obstacles one by one – and don't forget to check that you still want to get where you are heading.

Settle for the second-best clothes, car and home – but never settle for a second-best you.

# The stream always defeats the rock in the end, and it does so through perseverance.

Very few things that are truly worth having come to us easily. If you want them, you have to dare to take a risk.

# We may not all live holy lives, but we live in a world alive with holy moments.

*Kent Nerburn*

No real power can be given to you or taken from you. Ultimately, all power comes from within you.

How you treat those you think can do nothing for you determines the kind of person you really are.

**There is no more powerful phrase in the English language than 'thank you'.**

When a question is posed with humility, the universe tends to respond.

Life's battles don't always go
To the stronger or faster man,
But sooner or later the man who
wins. Is the one who thinks he can.

*Walter D. Wintle*

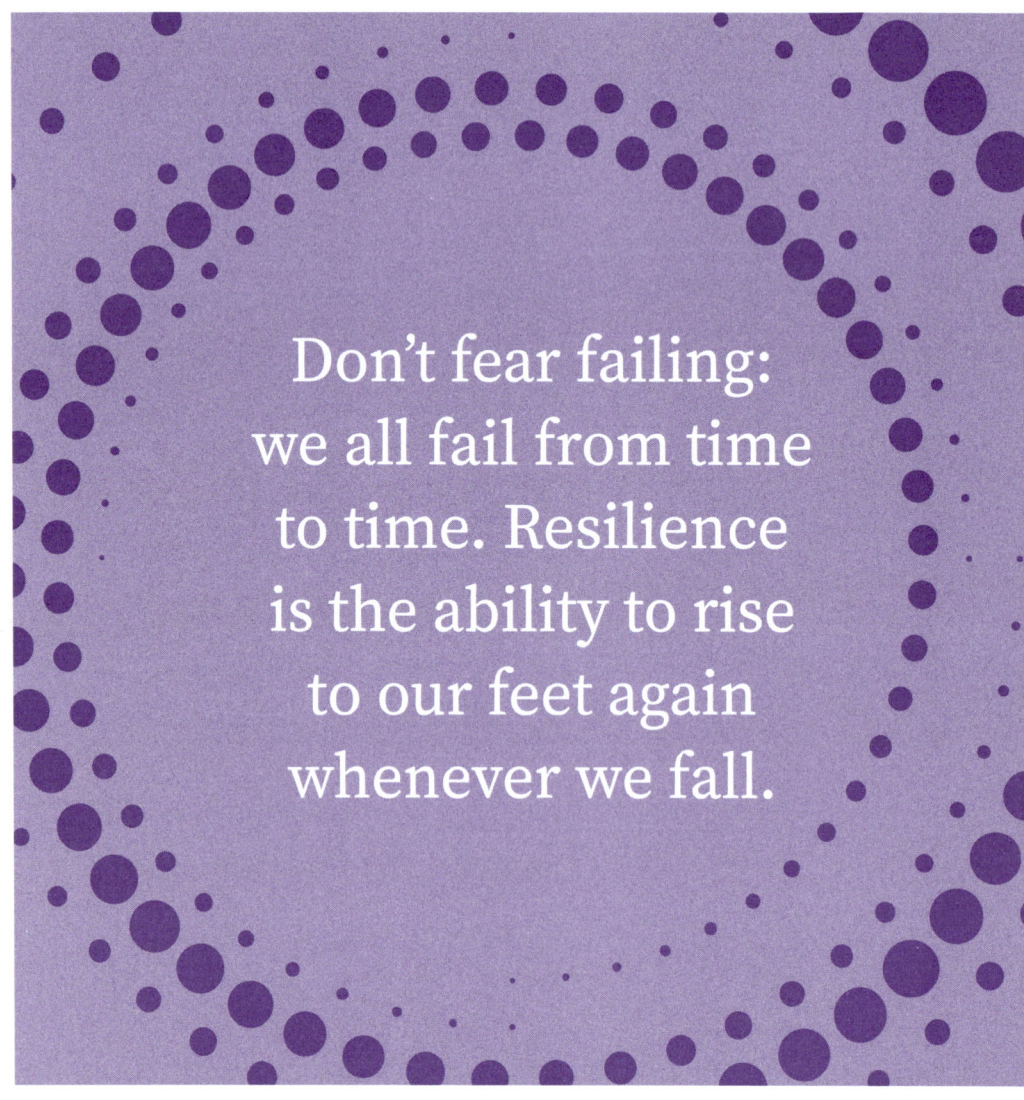

Don't fear failing: we all fail from time to time. Resilience is the ability to rise to our feet again whenever we fall.

Shakespeare once wrote that 'it is excellent to have a giant's strength, but tyrannous to use it like a giant'. The more power you have over others, the more you need to think about how to use that power responsibly.

Integrating the mind is the essence of life. Decide you will always say and do only what you feel is right. Then, you will come to tremendous clarity and conviction in the inner and outer worlds.

*Paramahamsa Nithyananda*

The way to develop a strong character is to always keep an open mind.

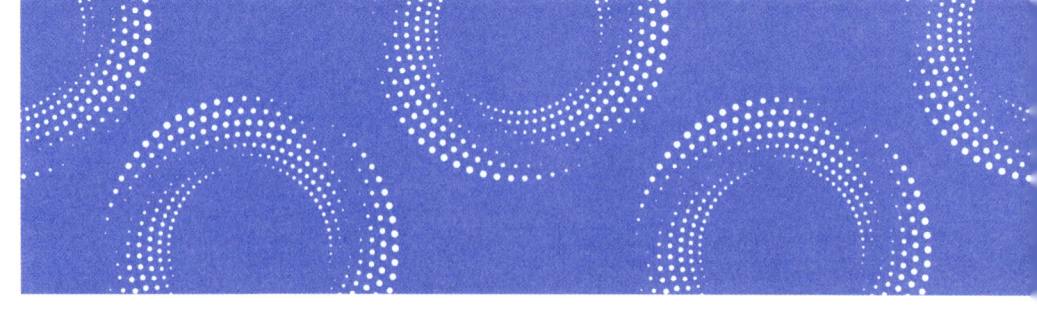

If you cannot find contentment within yourself, you will seek it in vain elsewhere.

Remember that what you do will always drown out what you say.

When our hatred is too bitter it places us below those whom we hate.

*François de La Rochefoucauld*

It's not enough to live. Resolve to live *for something*.

Any truth is better than indefinite doubt.

*Arthur Conan Doyle*

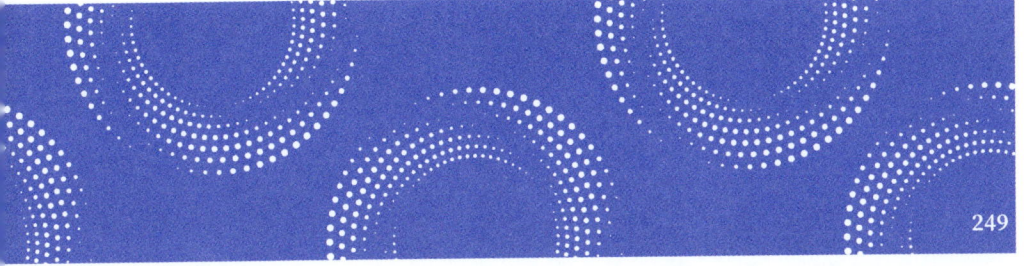

We sometimes spend so long preparing for the future that we are unprepared for the present.

**Aim to create happiness rather than find happiness: the more positivity you give, the more will come back to you.**

Just as a yacht would never get anywhere without the wind, so we would never get anywhere without change. The trick is to sail with the wind, not against it.

The cave you
fear to enter holds
the treasure you seek.
*Joseph Campbell*

**Nothing in life is ever
truly finished – and
that includes you.**

It is impossible to feel strong when you feel as though you are drifting. And it is impossible to feel weak once you have a clear sense of what your mission in life is.

**Just surviving isn't enough: the empowered person concentrates on thriving.**

Though you can fool others a lot of the time, you can never, ever fool yourself.

Your friends' enemies need not necessarily be your enemies.

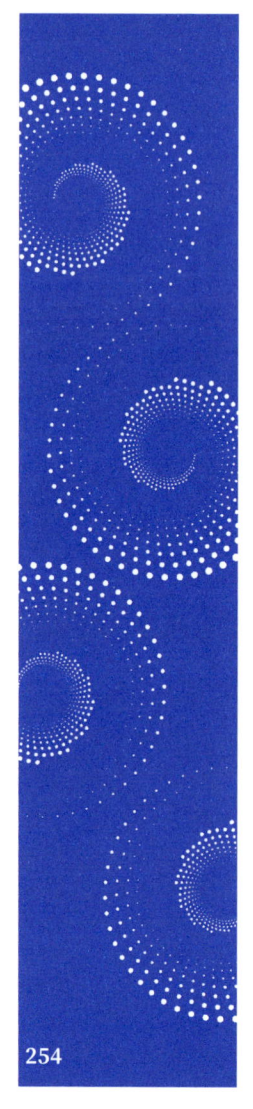

Health is the greatest possession. Contentment is the greatest treasure. Confidence is the greatest friend. Non-being is the greatest joy.
*Lao Tzu*

Peace comes from within. Do not look for it anywhere else.

Every significant
change begins by
fearlessly asking
'What if?'

If you have hope, and
humanity, and refuse
to sacrifice either, you
already have the power
to change the world.

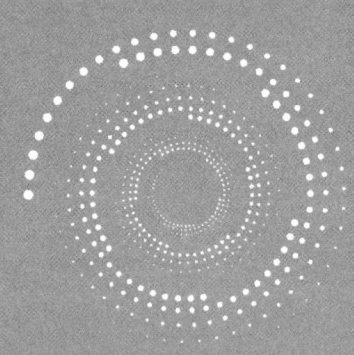

# The Guides

Words of advice, and warning, from those who have discovered the secrets of contentment – and others who have sought the secrets in vain.

Stretching his hand up to reach the stars, too often man forgets the flowers at his feet. *Jeremy Bentham*

**It is not length of life, but depth of life.**
*Ralph Waldo Emerson*

No matter what age you are, or what your circumstances might be, you are special, and you still have something unique to offer. Your life, because of who you are, has meaning.
*Barbara De Angelis*

Nobody can make you feel inferior without your consent. *Eleanor Roosevelt*

I may not have gone where I intended to go, but I think I have ended up where I needed to be. *Douglas Adams*

*If you want to conquer the anxiety of life, live in the moment, live in the breath.*
*Amit Ray*

**Always do whatever's next.**
*George Carlin*

Love is what we were born with.
Fear is what we learned here.
*Marianne Williamson*

Act as if what you do makes a
difference. It does.
*William James*

**The ultimate measure of a man is not where he stands in moments of comfort and convenience, but where he stands at times of challenge and controversy.**

*Martin Luther King, Jr.*

My religion is to live and die without regret.

*Milarepa*

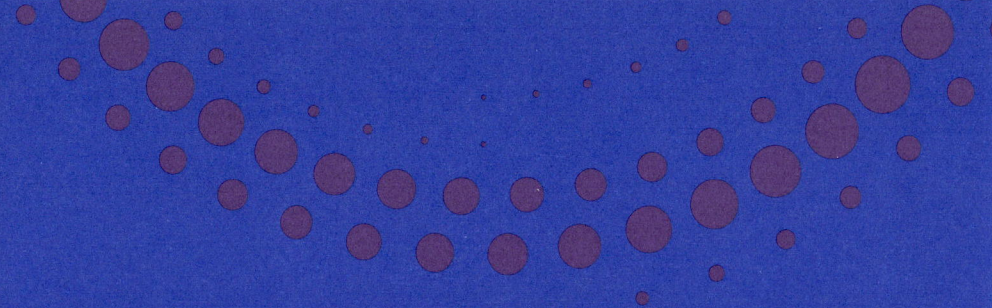

The thing that is really hard, and really amazing, is giving up on being perfect and beginning the work of becoming yourself.

*Anna Quindlen*

**Anxiety is something that is part of me, but it is not who I am.**

*Emma Stone*

# Sometimes even to live is an act of courage.

*Seneca the Younger*

If you realize that all things change, there is nothing you will try to hold on to. If you are not afraid of dying, there is nothing you cannot achieve.

*Lao Tzu*

Avoiding danger is no safer in the long run than outright exposure. The fearful are caught as often as the bold.
*Helen Keller*

Expect problems and eat them for breakfast.
*Alfred A. Montapert*

Households, cities, countries, and nations have enjoyed great happiness when a single individual has taken heed of the Good and Beautiful. Such people not only liberate themselves; they fill those they meet with a free mind.

*Philo*

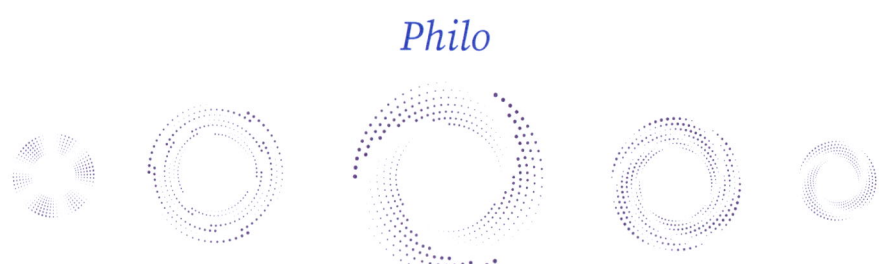

If we don't take charge of life's direction, our life will be controlled by the outside to serve the purpose of some other agency.

*Mihaly Csikszentmihalyi*

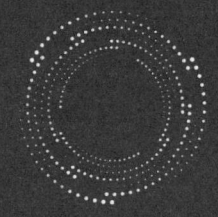

If I could give you one key,
and one key only, to more abundant life,
I would give you a sense of your own
worth, an unshakeable sense of your
own dignity as one grounded in the
source of the cosmic dance, as one
who plays a unique part in the unfolding
of the story of the world.

*Greta Crosby*

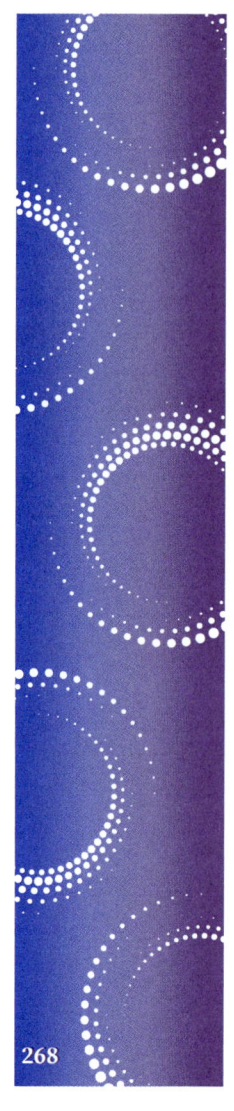

Our duty is to be useful, not according to our desires but according to our powers.

*Henri-Frédéric Amiel*

---

**We can draw lessons from the past, but we cannot live in it.**

*Lyndon B. Johnson*

Nothing great in the world has ever been accomplished without passion.

*Georg Wilhelm Friedrich Hegel*

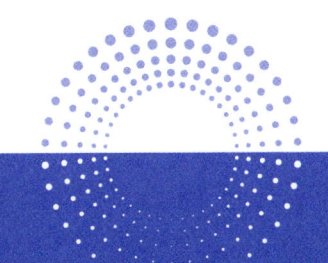

The most courageous act is still to think for yourself. Aloud.

*Coco Chanel*

The very least you can do in your life is to figure out what you hope for. And the most you can do is live inside that hope. Not admire it from a distance but live right in it, under its roof.

*Barbara Kingsolver*

**Be miserable.
Or motivate yourself.
Whatever has to be done,
it's always your choice.**

*Wayne Dyer*

Too many people are thinking of
security instead of opportunity.
They seem to be more afraid
of life than death.

*James F. Byrnes*

The trouble with
life isn't that there
is no answer, it's that
there are so many answers.

*Ruth Fulton Benedict*

All life is a chance. So take it! The person who goes furthest is the one who is willing to do and dare.

*Dale Carnegie*

Life is just a chance to grow a soul.

*A. Powell Davies*

# Excellence means when a man or woman asks of himself more than others do.

*José Ortega y Gasset*

I cannot believe that the purpose of life is to be 'happy'. I think the purpose of life is to be useful, to be responsible, to be compassionate. It is, above all, to matter and to count, to stand for something, to have made some difference that you lived at all.

*Leo C. Rosten*

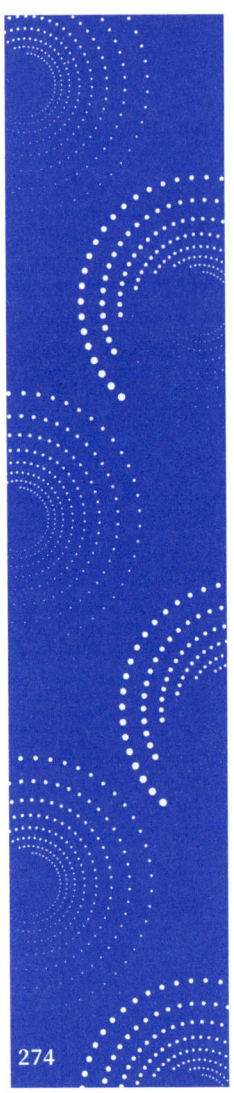

We can continue to try and clean up the gutters all over the world and spend all of our resources looking at just the dirty spots and trying to make them clean. Or we can lift our eyes up and look into the skies and move forward in an evolutionary way.

*Buzz Aldrin*

---

**Divide each difficulty into as many parts as is feasible and necessary to resolve it.**

*René Descartes*

One cannot say it too often:
There is nothing more prolific
in marvels than the art of
being free: but there is
nothing harder than the
apprenticeship of freedom.
*Alexis de Tocqueville*

I wish that every human life might
be pure transparent freedom.
*Simone de Beauvoir*

The harder
the conflict, the more
glorious the triumph.
*Thomas Paine*

A man who dares to waste
one hour of time has
not discovered the
value of life.
*Charles Darwin*

Those who have virtue always in their mouths, and neglect it in practice, are like a harp, which emits a sound pleasing to others, while itself is insensible of the music.

*Diogenes*

Love doesn't make the world go round; love is what makes the ride worthwhile.

*Franklin P. Jones*

The worst evil of all is to leave the ranks of the living before one dies.
*Seneca the Younger*

---

I don't want to get to the end of my life
and find that I lived just the length of it.
I want to have lived the width of it as well.
*Diane Ackerman*

---

**The mind is its own place, and in itself can make a heaven of hell, a hell of heaven.**
*John Milton*

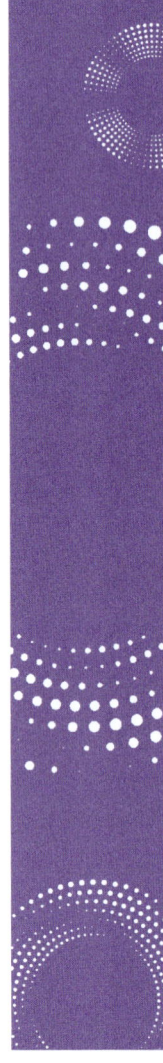

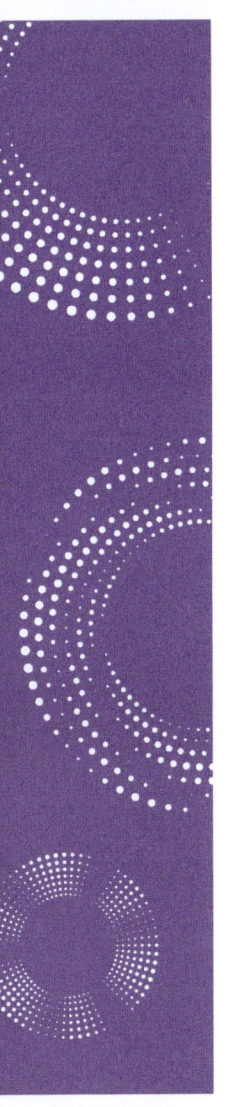

Unless you try to do something beyond what you have already mastered, you will never grow.
*Ronald E. Osborn*

Talk to yourself like you would to someone you love.
*Brené Brown*

As we are liberated from our own fear, our presence automatically liberates others.
*Marianne Williamson*

Strength does not come from winning.
Your struggles develop your strength.
When you go through hardship and decide
not to surrender, that is strength.
*Arnold Schwarzenegger*

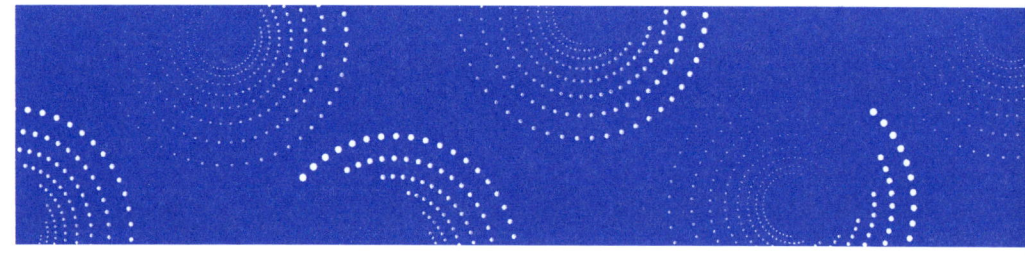

I know of no more encouraging
fact than the unquestionable
ability of man to elevate his life by
conscious endeavor.
*Henry David Thoreau*

Always go with the choice that scares you the most, because that's the one that is going to require the most from you. *Caroline Myss*

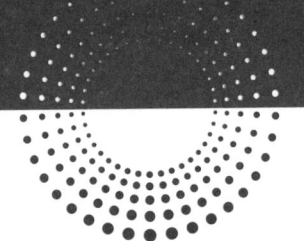

**The most difficult thing is the decision to act, the rest is merely tenacity.**
*Amelia Earhart*

**To change one's life:**

**1) Start immediately.**

**2) Do it flamboyantly.**

**3) No exceptions.**

*William James*

Success seems to be largely a matter of hanging on after others have let go.
*William Feather*

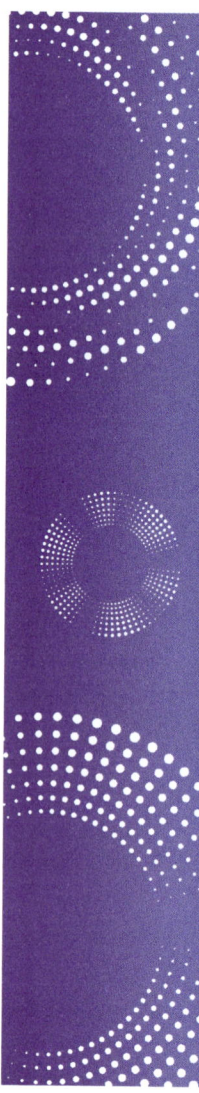

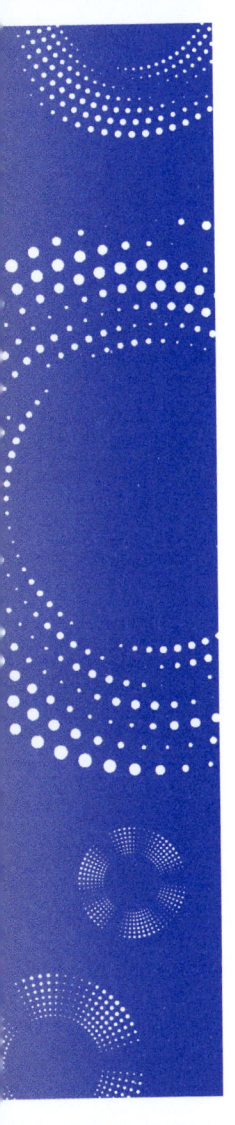

Expecting is the greatest impediment to living. In anticipation of tomorrow, it loses today.
*Seneca the Younger*

Imagination was given to man to compensate him for what he is not; a sense of humour to console him for what he is.
*Francis Bacon*

I cannot conceive of a good life which isn't, in some sense, a self-disciplined life.

*Philip Toynbee*

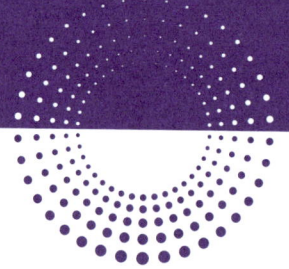

The cause of all our personal problems and nearly all the problems of the world can be summed up in a single sentence: human life is very deep, and our modern dominant lifestyle is not.

*Bo Lozoff*

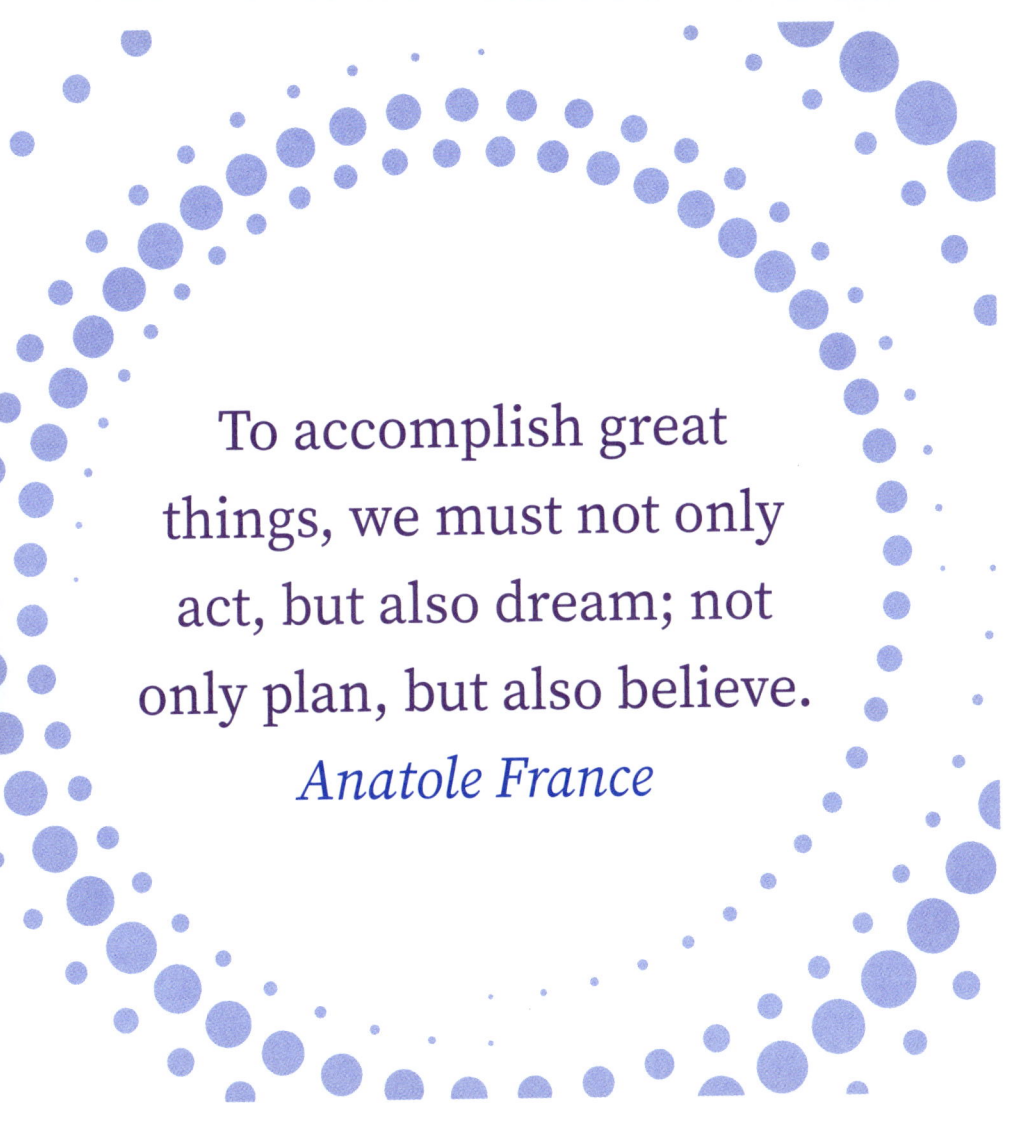

To accomplish great
things, we must not only
act, but also dream; not
only plan, but also believe.
*Anatole France*

Your own mind is a sacred enclosure
into which nothing harmful can
enter except by your permission.

*Arnold Bennett*

**Your own words are the**

**bricks and mortar of the**

**dreams you want to realize.**

**Your words are the greatest power**

**you have. The words you choose and**

**their use establish the life you experience.**

*Sonia Choquette*

**Experience is how life catches up with us and teaches us to love and forgive each other.**
*Judy Collins*

Once you say you're going to settle for second, that's what happens to you in life.
*John F. Kennedy*

Learn from the past, set vivid, detailed goals for the future, and live in the only moment of time over which you have any control: now. *Denis Waitley*

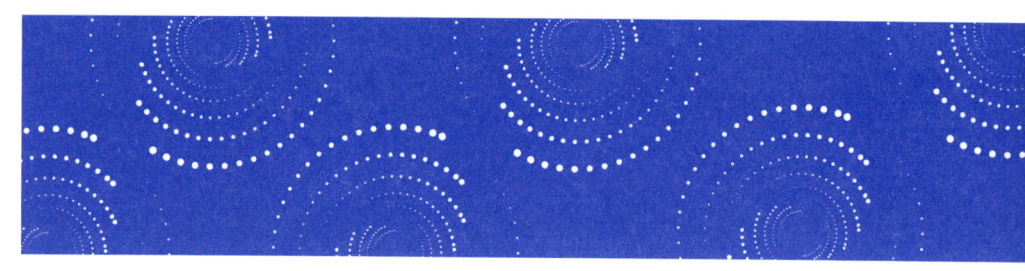

Where the willingness is great, the difficulties cannot be great. *Niccolò Machiavelli*

Life is meaningless only if we allow it to be.
Each of us has the power to give life meaning,
to make our time and our bodies and our words
into instruments of love and hope.

*Tom Head*

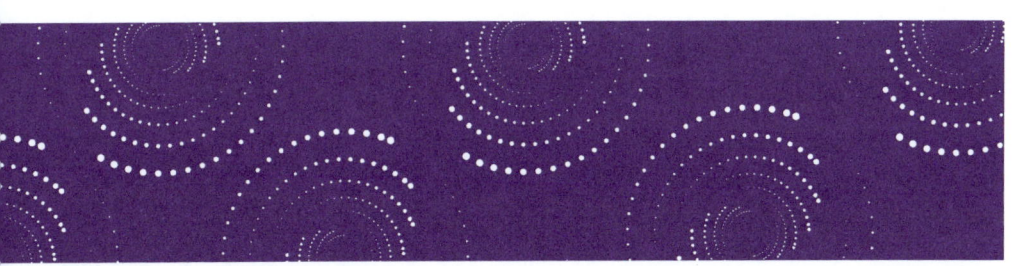

Life is just a quick succession of
busy nothings.

*Jane Austen*

In preparing
for battle I have always
found that plans are
useless, but planning
is indispensable.

*Dwight D. Eisenhower*

**If you ask me what I came into this life to do, I will tell you: I came to live out loud.**
*Émile Zola*

Without some goal and some effort to reach it, no one can live.
*Fyodor Dostoyevsky*

**Rules for happiness: something to do, someone to love, something to hope for.**
*Immanuel Kant*

I believe every human has a finite number of heartbeats. I don't intend to waste any of mine.
*Neil Armstrong*

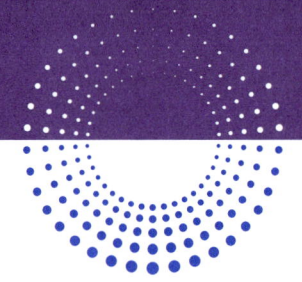

To be what we are, and to become what we are capable of becoming, is the only end of life.
*Robert Louis Stevenson*

# Problems are not stop signs, they are guidelines.
*Robert H. Schuller*

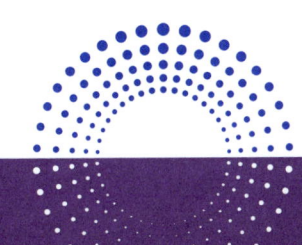

You desire to know the art of living, my friend? It is contained in one phrase: make use of suffering.

*Henri-Frédéric Amiel*

Things turn out best for the people who make the best out of the way things turn out.
*Art Linkletter*

**The object in life is not to be on the side of the majority, but to escape finding oneself in the ranks of the insane.**
*Marcus Aurelius*

Gratefulness is the key to a happy life that we hold in our hands, because if we are not grateful, then no matter how much we have we will not be happy – because we will always want to have something else or something more.

*David Steindl-Rast*

**Set your sights high, the higher the better. Expect the most wonderful things to happen, not in the future but right now. Realize that nothing is too good. Allow absolutely nothing to hamper you or hold you up in any way.**

*Eileen Caddy*

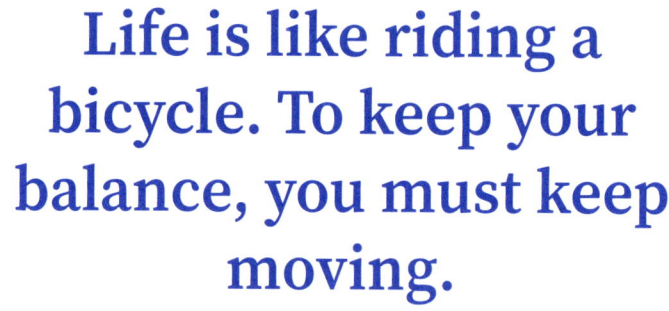

**Life is like riding a bicycle. To keep your balance, you must keep moving.**
*Albert Einstein*

Nothing else matters much
– not wealth, nor learning, nor
even health – without this gift: the
spiritual capacity to keep zest in
living. This is the creed of creeds,
the final deposit and distillation
of all important faiths: that you
should be able to believe in life.

*Harry Emerson Fosdick*

Fortune favours the bold. *Virgil*

If you want to improve, be content to be thought foolish and stupid. *Epictetus*

A journey of a thousand miles must begin with a single step. *Lao Tzu*

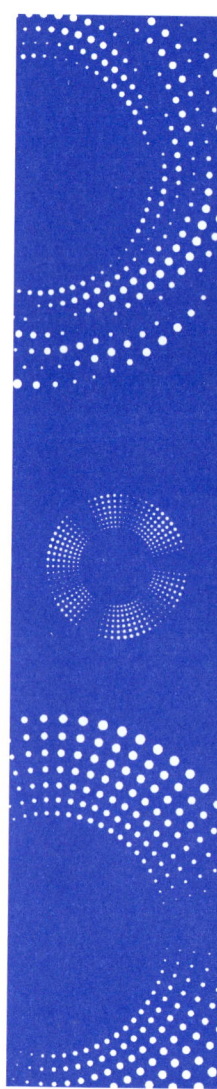

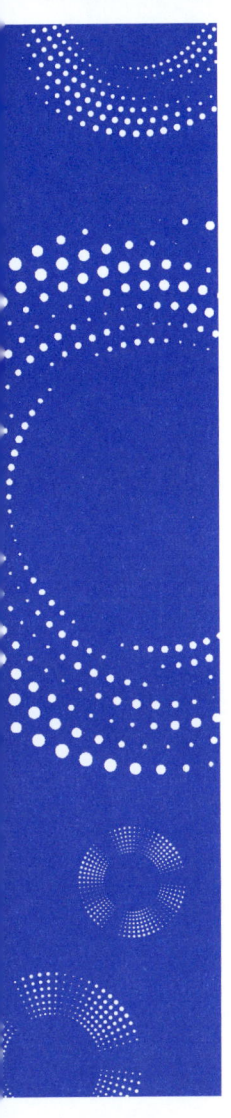

# What do we live for, if it is not to make life less difficult for each other?

*George Eliot*

---

Achievement seems to be connected with action. Successful men and women keep moving. They make mistakes, but they don't quit.

*Conrad Hilton*

---

Surround yourself with only people who are going to lift you higher.

*Oprah Winfrey*

How far you go in life depends on your being tender with the young, compassionate with the aged, sympathetic with the striving, and tolerant of the weak and strong. Because some day in life you will have been all of these.

*George Washington Carver*

Life can only be understood backwards; but it must be lived forwards.

*Søren Kierkegaard*

Many will call me an adventurer –
and that I am, only one of a different
sort: one of those who risks his
skin to prove his platitudes.

*Che Guevara*

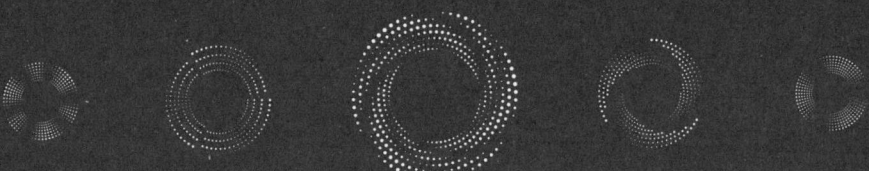

Isn't it a noble, an enlightened way of spending our
brief time in the sun, to work at understanding the
universe and how we have come to wake up in it? This
is how I answer when I am asked – as I am surprisingly
often – why I bother to get up in the mornings.

*Richard Dawkins*

I've learned that you shouldn't go through life with a catcher's mitt on both hands; you need to be able to throw something back.
*Maya Angelou*

That it will never come again is what makes life so sweet.
*Emily Dickinson*

If you want to be happy, set a goal that commands your thoughts, liberates your energy, and inspires your hopes.
*Andrew Carnegie*

Be slow to fall into friendship; but when thou art in, continue firm and constant.

*Socrates*

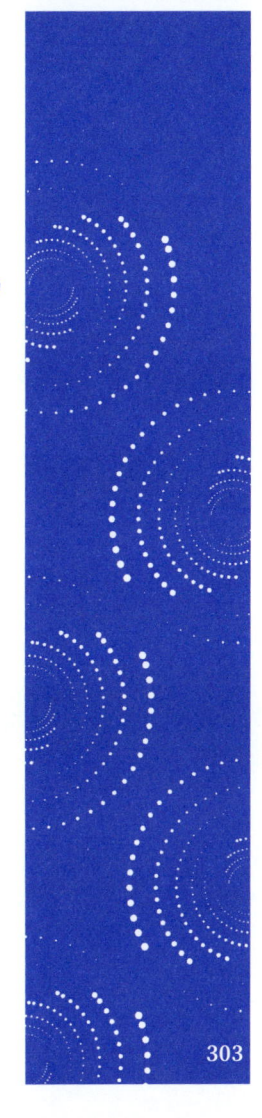

# If a victory is told in detail, one can no longer distinguish it from a defeat.

*Jean-Paul Sartre*

There is a fountain of youth: it is your mind, your talents, the creativity you bring to your life and the lives of people you love. When you learn to tap this source, you will truly have defeated age.

*Sophia Loren*

Hope is the only good that is common to all men; those who have nothing else possess hope still.
*Thales of Miletus*

All men have a sweetness in their life. That is what helps them go on. It is towards that they turn when they feel too worn out.
*Albert Camus*

Leap, and the net will appear. *John Burroughs*

**There is only one way to happiness and that is to cease worrying about things which are beyond the power of our will.** *Epictetus*

It is only when we truly know and understand that we have a limited time on Earth and that we have no way of knowing when our time is up that we will begin to live each day to the fullest, as if it were the only one we had. *Elisabeth Kübler-Ross*

**The love we have in our youth is superficial compared to the love that an old man has for his old wife.** *Will Durant*

# May you live every day of your life.
*Jonathan Swift*

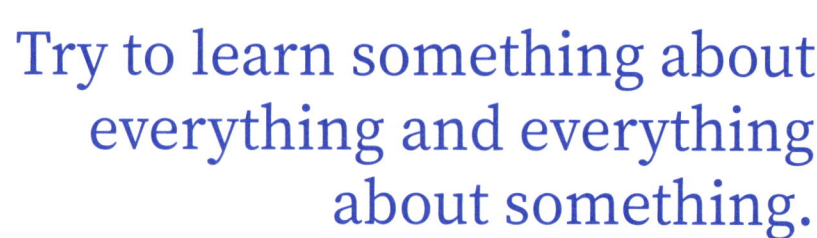

Try to learn something about everything and everything about something.
*Thomas Huxley*

**There is only one day left, always starting over: it is given to us at dawn and taken away from us at dusk.**
*Jean-Paul Sartre*

The error of youth is to believe that intelligence is a substitute for experience, while the error of age is to believe experience is a substitute for intelligence.
*Ernest Hemingway*

The young do not know enough to be prudent, and therefore they attempt the impossible – and achieve it, generation after generation.

*Pearl S. Buck*

Always concentrate on how far you have come, rather than how far you have left to go. The difference in how easy it seems will amaze you.

*Heidi Johnson*

You can discover more about a person in an hour of play than in a year of conversation.
*Plato*

Life is mostly froth and bubble; Two things stand like stone: Kindness in another's trouble, Courage in our own.
*Adam Gordon*

We are just an advanced breed
of monkeys on a minor planet
of a very average star. But we
can understand the Universe.
That makes us something
very special.
*Stephen Hawking*

Keep true to the dreams
of your youth.
*Friedrich von Schiller*

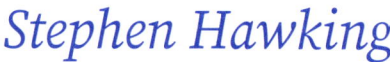

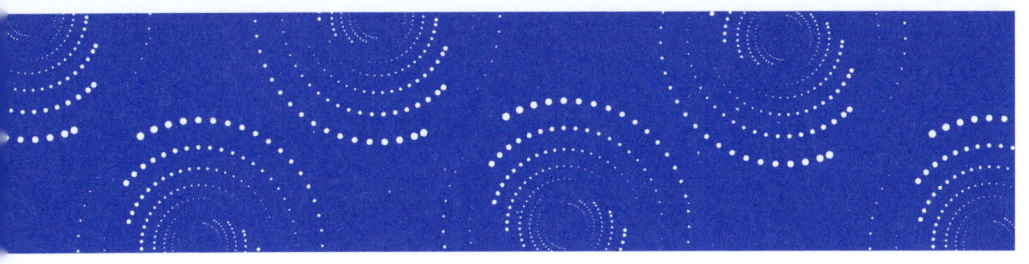

Hope is both the earliest and the most indispensable virtue inherent in the state of being alive. If life is to be sustained hope must remain, even where confidence is wounded, trust impaired.

*Erik H. Erikson*

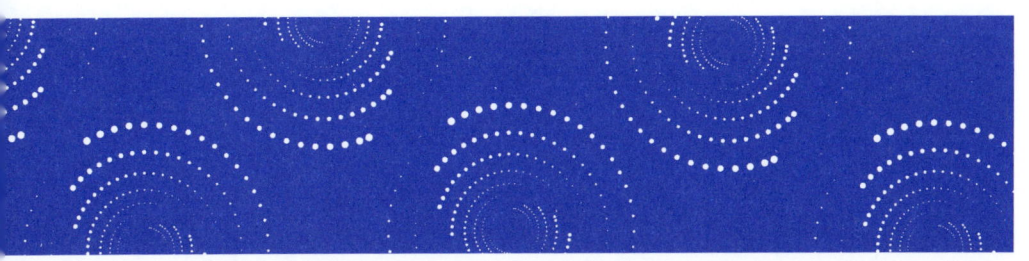

The first requisite of success is the ability to apply your physical and mental energies to one problem without growing weary.

*Thomas Edison*

An idea is never given to you without you being given the power to make it reality. You must, nevertheless, suffer for it.

*Richard Bach*

Friendship improves happiness and abates misery by the doubling of our joy and the dividing of our grief.

*Marcus Cicero*

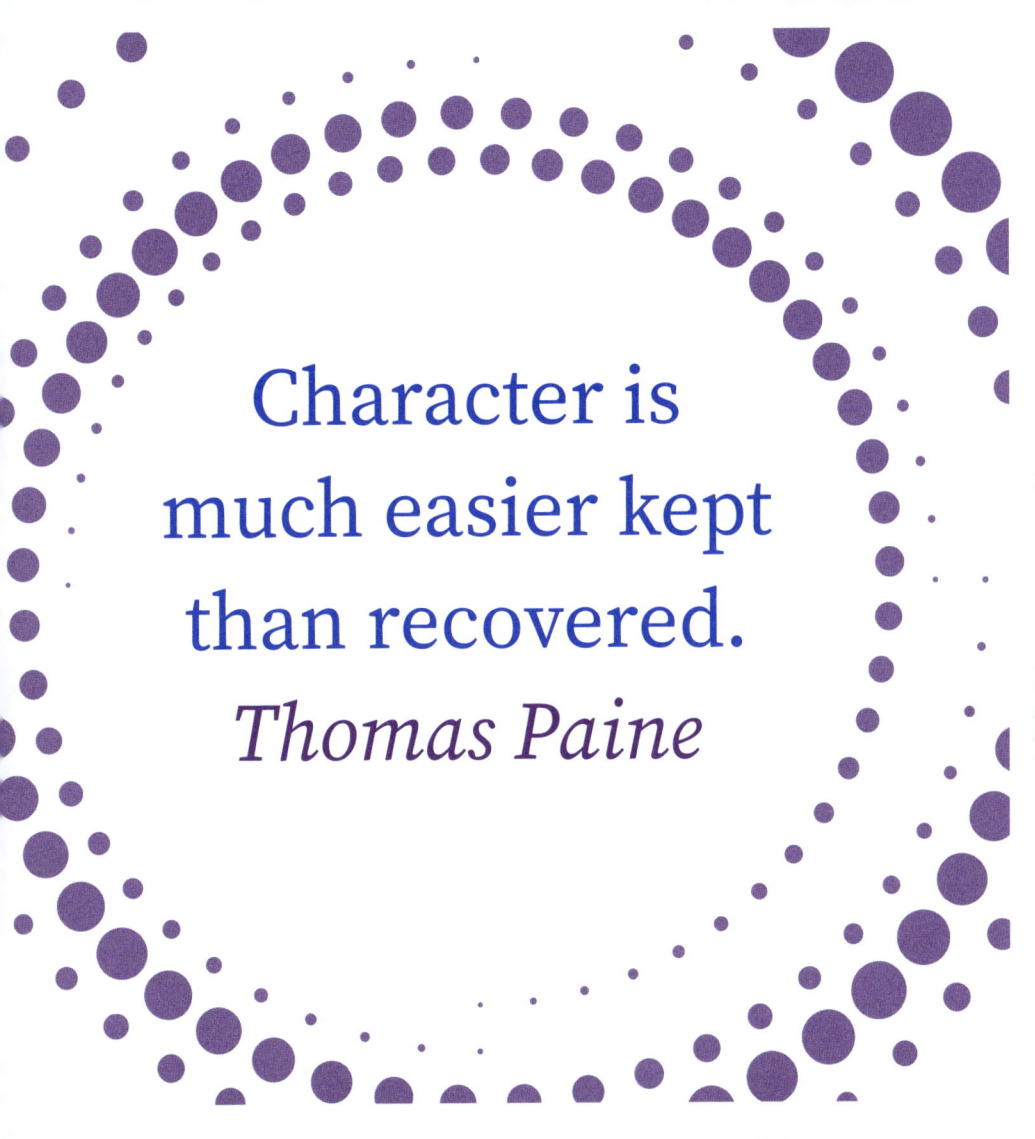

Character is
much easier kept
than recovered.
*Thomas Paine*

Nothing is so difficult as not deceiving oneself.
*Ludwig Wittgenstein*

Who is happy? A person who has a healthy body, is dowered with peace of mind, and cultivates his talents.
*Thales of Miletus*

Do not look back on happiness or dream of it in the future. You are only sure of today; do not let yourself be cheated of it.
*Henry Ward Beecher*

**The question isn't who's going to let me; it's who is going to stop me.**
*Ayn Rand*

Don't be afraid of the space between your dreams and reality. If you can dream it, you can make it so.
*Belva Davis*

Faith is taking the first step even when you don't see the whole staircase.
*Martin Luther King, Jr.*

The difference between those who succeed and those who fail isn't what they have – it's what they choose to see and do with their resources and their expertise of life.
*Anthony Robbins*

---

**I'd rather regret the things I've done than regret the things I haven't done.**
*Lucille Ball*

Anxiety is like a rocking chair. It gives you something to do, but it doesn't get you very far. *Jodi Picoult*

That so few now dare to be eccentric marks the chief danger of our time. *John Stuart Mill*

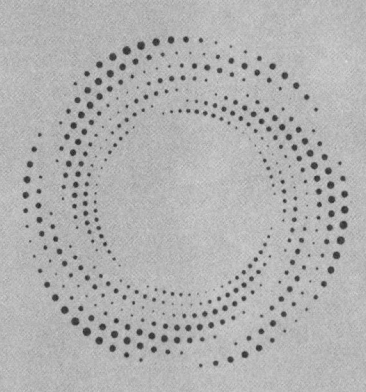

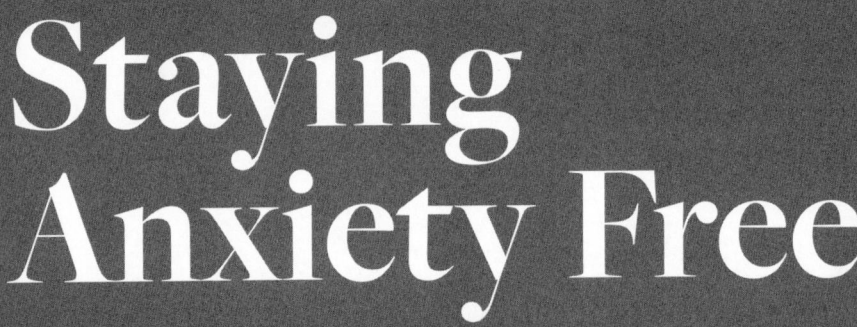

# Staying Anxiety Free

It is easy to feel calm when things are going well, but how do we remain serene in the face of setbacks? In this section we explore how to feel resilient when we most need it – in times of trouble.

Give yourself permission to feel low:
we all feel a little defeated by life
at times. How would we know how
precious happiness is if we had never
known anything else?

All difficult things have their origin in that which is easy, and great things in that which is small.

*Lao Tzu*

Most people give up when they are frustrated, rather than exhausted. Give yourself a change of scene, and force yourself to laugh at your frustrations – they will soon then fade away.

When you organize and eliminate clutter, you free yourself from stress and anxiety by eliminating feelings of overwhelm.
*S. J. Scott*

Troubles melt away when faced bravely with all your inner strength.

Not everything you face in life can be changed, but you can change nothing until you have faced it.

When you get into a tight place and everything goes against you, till it seems as though you could not hold on a minute longer, never give up then, for that is just the place and time that the tide will turn.
*Harriet Beecher Stowe*

**When things go wrong, remember that nothing is as valuable as experience.**

**It may be that when we no longer know what to do, we have come to our real work, and when we no longer know which way to go, we have begun our real journey.**
*Wendell Berry*

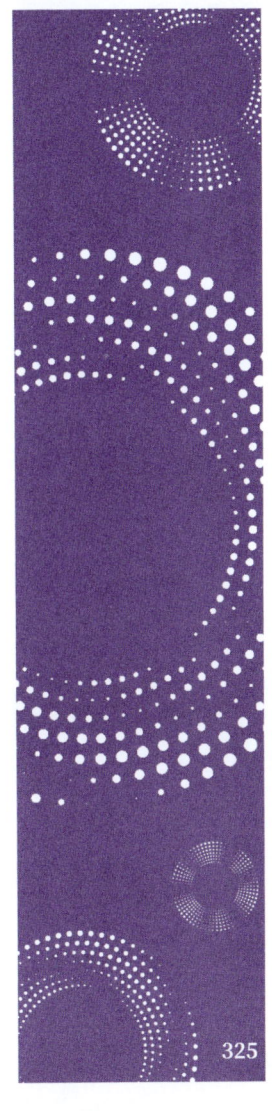

Stay strong: Albert Einstein was told he would 'never amount to much' by his teachers. He paid no attention to their criticism, and ended up doing relatively well . . .

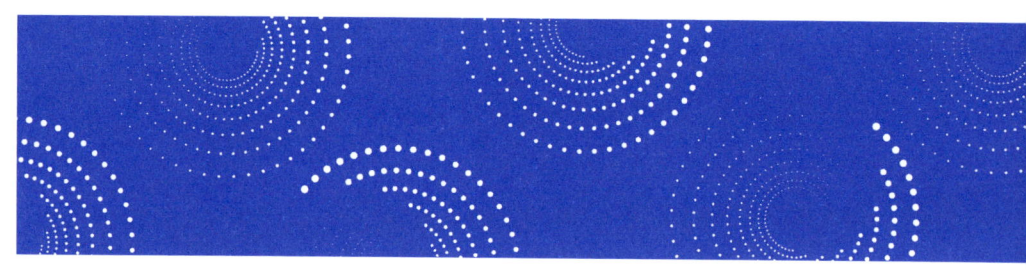

Almost everything will work again if you unplug it for a few minutes, including you. *Anne Lamott*

Deep down we all know there is truth in the saying that 'the best things in life are free'. Why, then, do we so often forget to enjoy the tremendous riches that lie all around us?

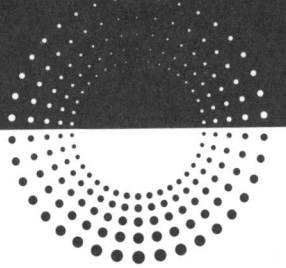

Nothing drains enthusiasm more rapidly than chasing at full speed down a path you do not really wish to follow. Check and recheck what you really want in life.

I've found, as a general rule of life, that the things you think are going to be the scariest nearly always turn out not so bad after all.

*P.G. Wodehouse*

**You cannot possess happiness: we do not talk of 'having' happiness, only of sometimes 'being' happy. So always aim to be, not to have.**

**Don't worry if you sometimes feel weak: courage is far more important than strength.**

A man can fail many times, but he isn't a failure until he begins to blame somebody else.
*John Burroughs*

**The quickest way to feel better is to help somebody else to feel better.**

Anyone who says only sunshine brings happiness has never danced in the rain.

As long as the world is turning and spinning, we're gonna be dizzy and we're gonna make mistakes.
*Mel Brooks*

Difficult circumstances reveal your true character.

There is a great deal to be said for wishful thinking, and even more to be said for wishful doing.

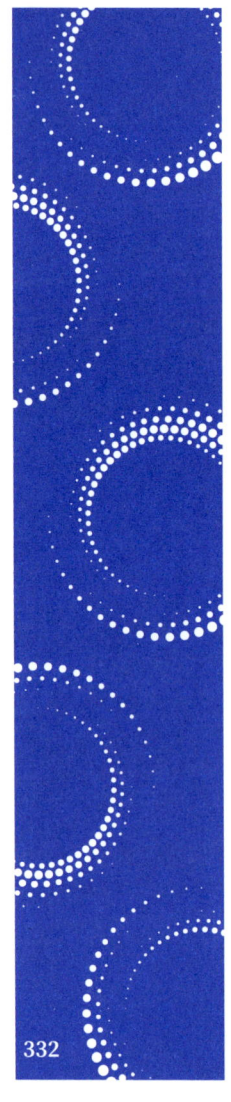

If you make giving up unthinkable, carrying on becomes the only possible thing to do.

So long as I am acting
from duty and conviction,
I am indifferent to taunts and
jeers. I think they
will probably do me
 more good than harm.

*Winston Churchill*

332

You don't always reap what you sow in this life – but don't let that stop you sowing goodness for others to reap.

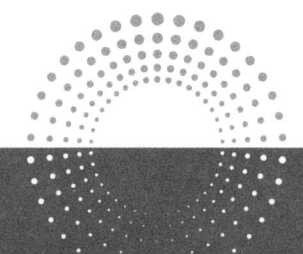

Even mighty buildings sometimes fall in the face of earthquakes. The buildings that survive are the ones that were designed to sway a little to absorb the shock.

Part of maturing into full adulthood involves unlearning the fears that were instilled within us in childhood.

Out of suffering have emerged the strongest souls; the most massive characters are seared with scars.

*Khalil Gibran*

The primary cause of unhappiness is not the situation, but your thoughts about it. Be aware of the thoughts you are thinking. Separate them from the situation, which is always neutral, which always is as it is.
*Eckhart Tolle*

You do not need armour to withstand life's blows: be open to others, but keep on your toes and develop quick reflexes.

**Rivers never hurry, and never panic. Yet they always reach the sea in the end.**

Now and then, loneliness is the price you pay for having convictions. It may hurt, but it is still a price worth paying.

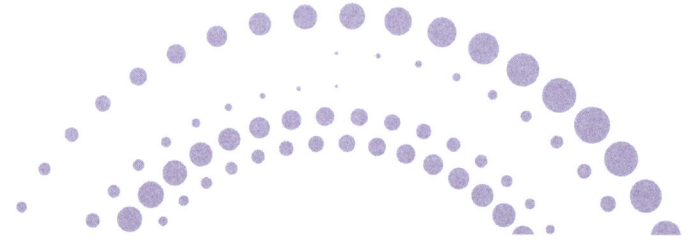

In order to feel good, you sometimes have to think positively and wait for your feelings to catch up with your thoughts.

He who is not everyday conquering some fear has not learned the secret of life.

*Ralph Waldo Emerson*

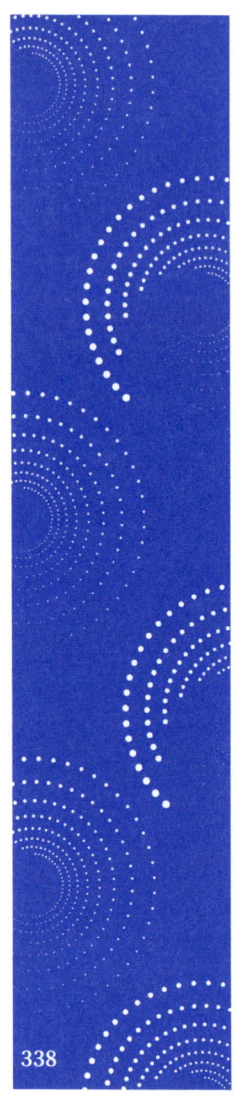

Ask yourself 'What's the worst that can happen?' Usually the answer is not nearly as frightening as you think.

For every failure, there's an alternative course of action. You just have to find it. When you come to a roadblock, take a detour.
*Mary Kay Ash*

Fear is only natural, like the vertigo many of us feel when standing at a cliff edge. All it tells us is that we're doing something dangerous – but sometimes doing something dangerous is exactly what we need to do.

The easy path ultimately leads nowhere: only overcoming difficulties creates true character.

Brick walls prevent your progress only if you try to walk through them. Find a way around them, or learn how to climb.

Inaction breeds doubt and fear. Action breeds confidence and courage. If you want to conquer fear, do not sit home and think about it. Go out and get busy.
*Dale Carnegie*

I myself am made entirely of flaws, stitched together with good intentions.

*Augusten Burroughs*

Take heart: the Beatles were initially turned down by Decca Recording Studios, who said 'We don't like their sound.' You'll get by with a little help from your friends.

To underestimate oneself is as much a departure from truth as to exaggerate one's own powers.
*Arthur Conan Doyle*

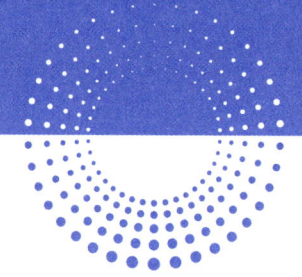

It is when the storm is at its fiercest that the world most needs its lighthouses: keep shining!

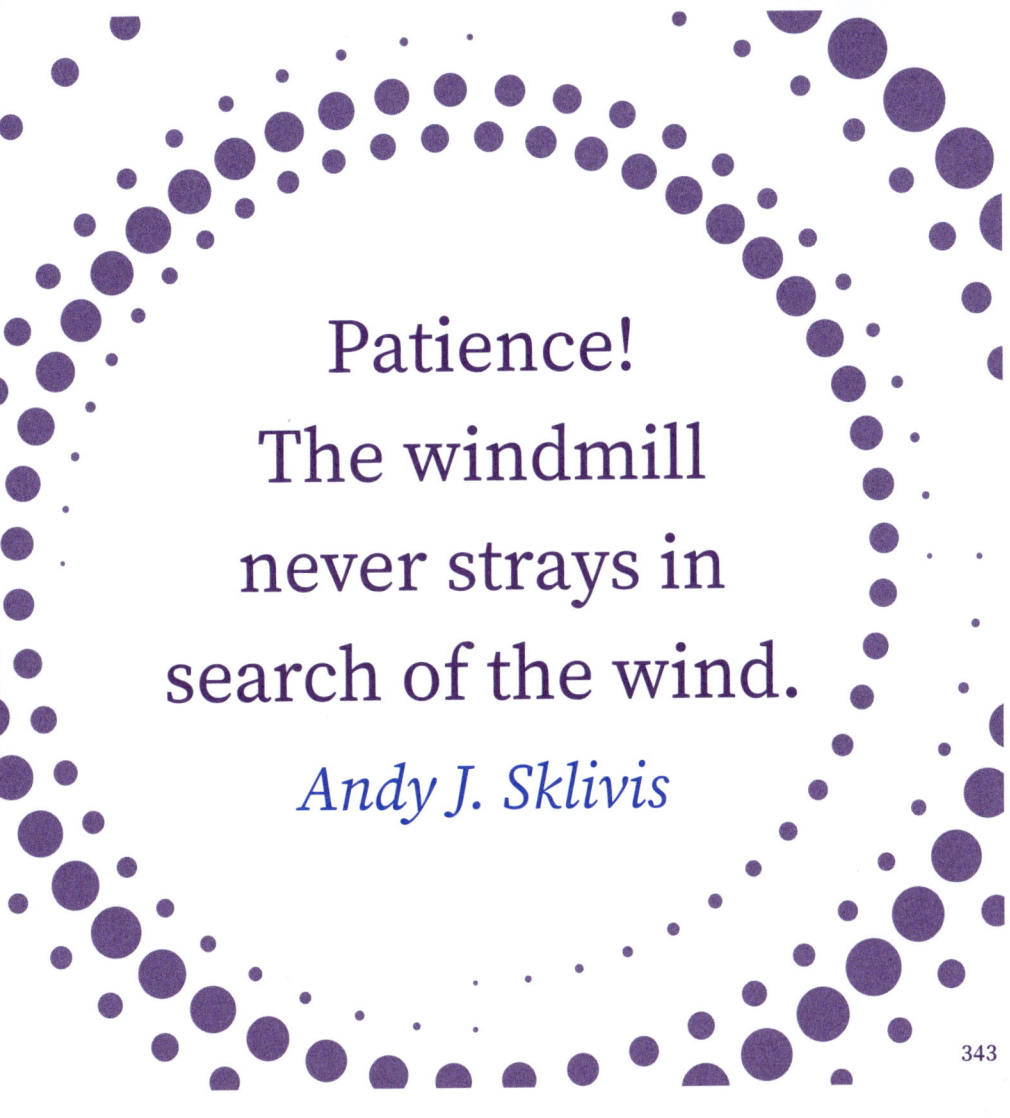

Patience!
The windmill
never strays in
search of the wind.

*Andy J. Sklivis*

Life is many things, but it is never boring. If you experience boredom, then you need to change the way you view the world.

Courage is not the absence of fear, but rather the judgement that something else is more important than fear.
*Ambrose Redmoon*

Don't throw in the towel –
dry your tears with it and try again.

# True faith in yourself is harder than diamonds.

Never give up: Walt Disney was once fired from a newspaper job for 'lacking imagination'. Turned out he wasn't such a Dumbo after all!

**Many of those who give up never realize that they did so on the very brink of success.**

Welcome each and every day as soon as you get out of bed in the morning.

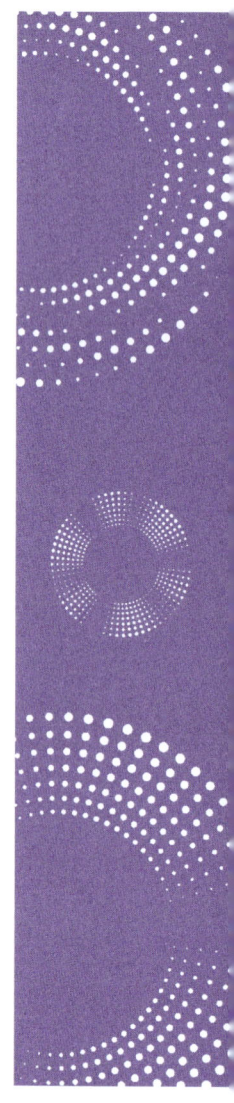

Most of the shadows of this life are caused by our standing in our own sunshine.
*Ralph Waldo Emerson*

**It is easy to blame others when things go wrong, but it is usually more productive to look at ourselves and how we might do better next time.**

Don't expect to always thrive: sometimes to simply endure is a type of victory.

**Sometimes the sanest thing to do is just wallow in the misery for a while. Then climb out, grab a towel, dry off, and go about living.**
*Kevin D. Weeks*

Success is not final, failure is not fatal – it is the courage to continue that counts.

*Winston Churchill*

If you're feeling low for long periods of time, consult your doctor. Remember that true depression is a flaw in chemistry, not in character.

Life is not what it's supposed to be. It's what it is. The way you cope with it is what makes the difference.

*Virginia Satir*

We would never develop our strengths if we had nothing to push against.

If something you have tried turns out to be impossible, then rejoice! Congratulations on finding the limits of what is possible. Now, if you back your dream up by just 1 per cent, you will see something that is extraordinary yet also achievable.

Sometimes you have to be flexible and yield in the face of life's pressures, but you should never be tempted to sacrifice your core values no matter what the world throws at you.

# The Power of Laughter

The truly happy can laugh at themselves. In this section we collect wit from throughout the ages and across the world to look at the lighter side of staying anxiety free.

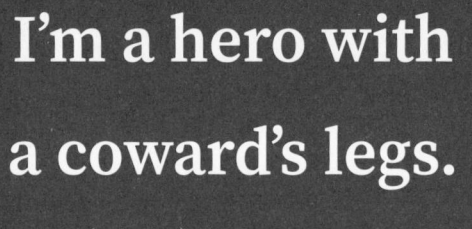

I'm a hero with
a coward's legs.

*Spike Milligan*

You grow up the day you have your first real laugh at yourself.
*Ethel Barrymore*

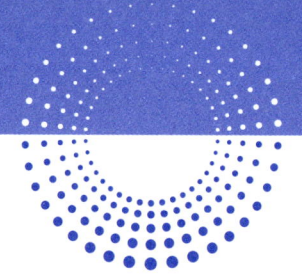

Don't go backwards, you have already been there.
*Ray Charles*

Before you marry a person, you should first make them use a computer with slow internet to see who they really are. *Will Ferrell*

**Sober or blotto, this is your motto: keep muddling through.** *P. G. Wodehouse*

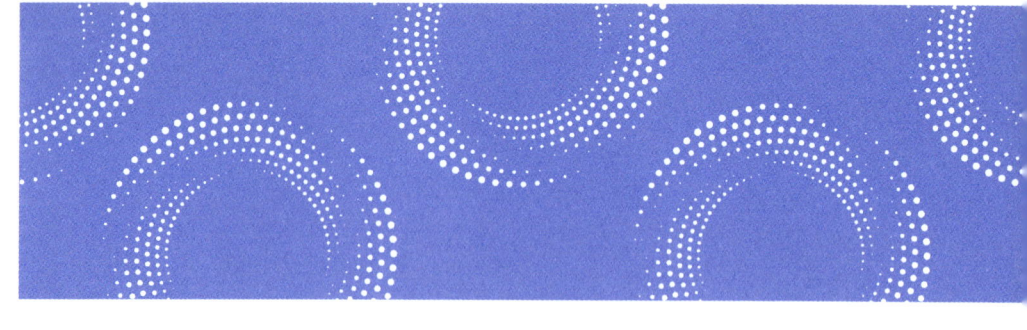

Fear is that little darkroom
where negatives are developed.
*Michael Pritchard*

**Some people never
go crazy. What
truly horrible lives
they must lead.**
*Charles Bukowski*

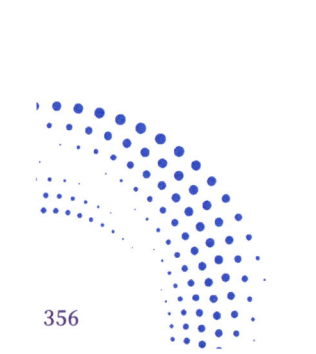

I like to think of my behavior in the Sixties as a 'learning experience'. Then again, I like to think of anything stupid I've done as a 'learning experience'. It makes me feel less stupid.

*P. J. O'Rourke*

It's not denial.
I'm just selective
about the reality I accept.
*Calvin and Hobbes*

**I'm sick of following my dreams. I'm just going to ask them where they're goin', and hook up with them later.**

*Mitch Hedberg*

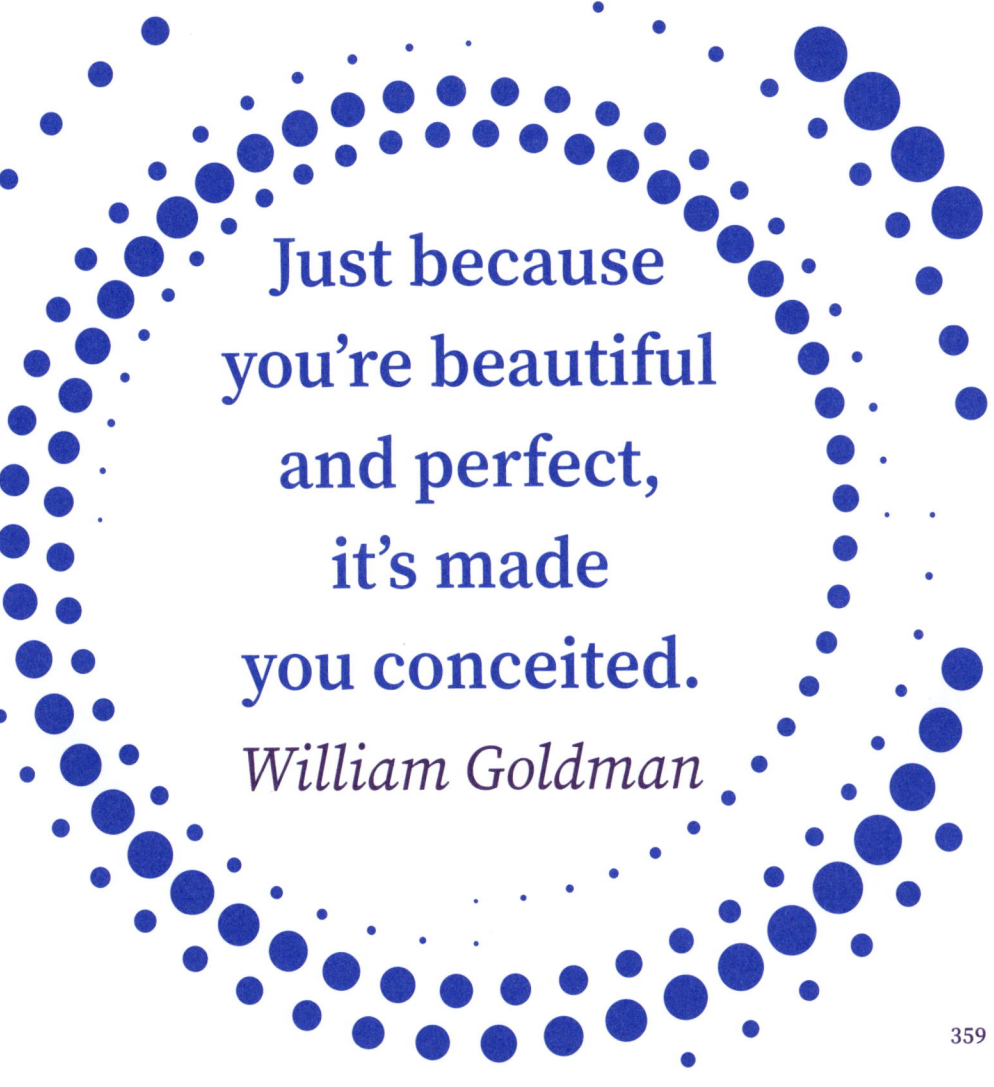

Just because
you're beautiful
and perfect,
it's made
you conceited.
*William Goldman*

Be like a postage stamp – stick to one thing until you get there.
*Josh Billings*

Opportunity does not knock, it presents itself when you beat down the door.
*Kyle Chandler*

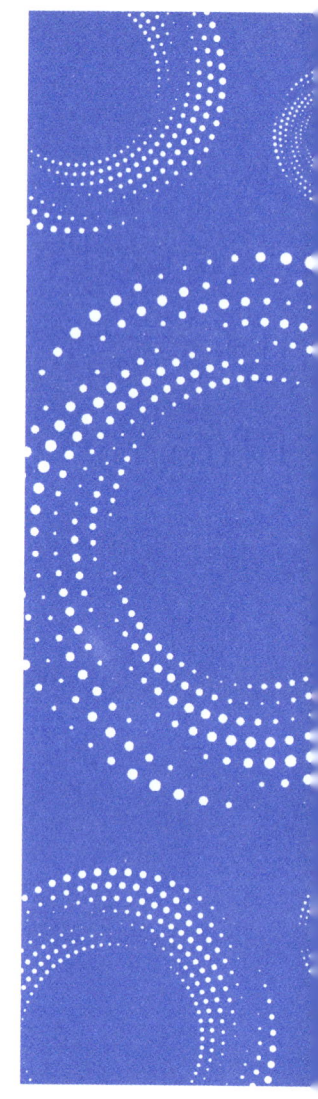

It's the good girls who
keep diaries, the bad girls
never have the time.
*Tallulah Bankhead*

Since everything is but
an apparition, having
nothing to do with good
or bad, acceptance or
rejection, one may
well burst out in laughter.
*Longchenpa*

It is easy for me to love myself, but for ladies to do it is another question altogether.

*Johnny Vegas*

Normal is getting dressed in clothes that you buy for work and driving through traffic in a car that you are still paying for – in order to get to the job you need to pay for the clothes and the car, and the house you leave vacant all day so you can afford to live in it.

*Ellen Goodman*

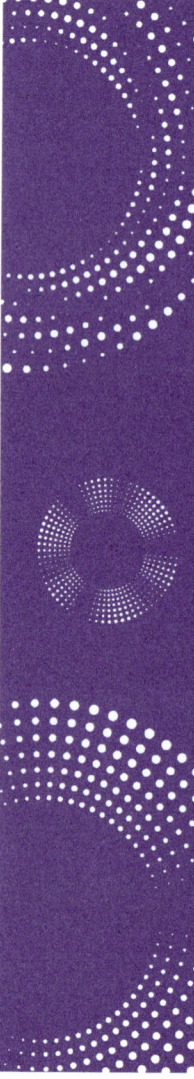

It is better to be roughly right than to be precisely wrong.
*John Maynard Keynes*

Always remember you're unique, just like everyone else.
*Alison Boulter*

As Shakespeare says, if you're going to do a thing you might as well pop right at it and get it over.
*P. G. Wodehouse*

If you think too long on your next step, you will end up in life standing on one leg.
*Chinese proverb*

My doctor says that I have a malformed public-duty gland and a natural deficiency in moral fibre and that I am therefore excused from saving universes. *Douglas Adams*

Just remember, when you're over the hill, you begin to pick up speed. *Charles M. Schulz*

Every cloud has its silver lining but it is sometimes a little difficult to get it to the mint.
*Don Marquis*

I used to think anyone doing anything weird was weird. Now I know that it is the people that call others weird that are weird.
*Paul McCartney*

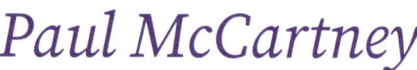

Stop wearing your wishbone where your backbone ought to be.

*Elizabeth Gilbert*

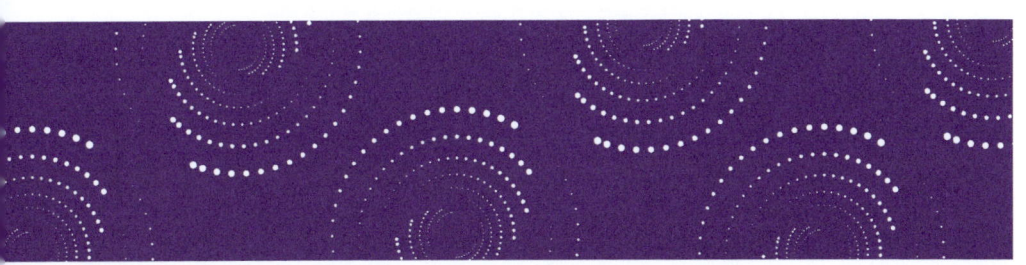

I can't go back to yesterday because I was a different person then.

*Lewis Carroll*

**Television connects viewers to nothing except the assumption of being connected to something.** *Michael Arlen*

**It ain't what they call you, it's what you answer to.** *W.C. Fields*

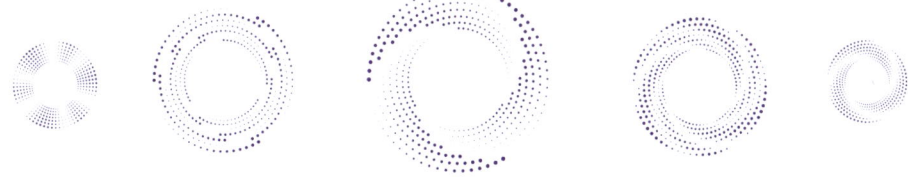

The problem is not that there are problems. The problem is expecting otherwise and thinking that having problems is a problem.

*Theodore Rubin*

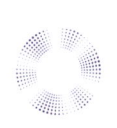
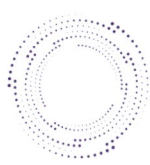
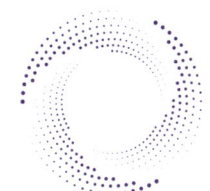
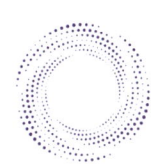
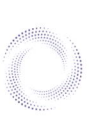

**It's not your job to like me, it's mine.**
*Byron Katie*

**In three words I can sum up everything I've learned about life: it goes on.**
*Robert Frost*

**Good judgment comes from experience. Experience comes from bad judgment.**
*Jim Horning*

**If you ask what is the single most important key to longevity, I would have to say it is avoiding worry, stress and tension. And if you didn't ask me, I'd still have to say it.**
*George F. Burns*

**Flattery is like cologne water, to be smelt, not swallowed.**
*Josh Billings*

---

I have not failed. I've just found 10,000 ways that won't work.
*Thomas Edison*

**If you obey all the rules, you miss all the fun.**

*Katharine Hepburn*

---

My uncle Sammy was an angry man. He had printed on his tombstone: 'What are you looking at?'

*Margaret Smith*

**Don't cry because it's over, smile because it happened.**
*Dr. Seuss*

My therapist told me the way to achieve true inner peace is to finish what I start. So far today, I have finished two bags of M&M's and a chocolate cake. I feel better already.

*Dave Barry*

It's a funny thing about life; if you refuse to accept anything but the best, you very often get it.

*W. Somerset Maugham*

Life isn't fair, it's just fairer than death, that's all.
*William Goldman*

The cure for boredom is curiosity. There is no cure for curiosity.
*Ellen Parr*

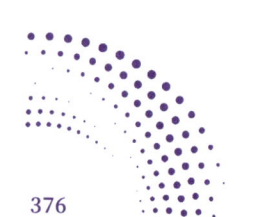

Advice is what we ask for when we already know the answer but wish we didn't.
*Erica Jong*

Most people work just hard enough not to get fired and get paid just enough money not to quit.

*George Carlin*

I have a simple philosophy: fill what's empty. Empty what's full. Scratch where it itches.

*Alice Roosevelt Longworth*

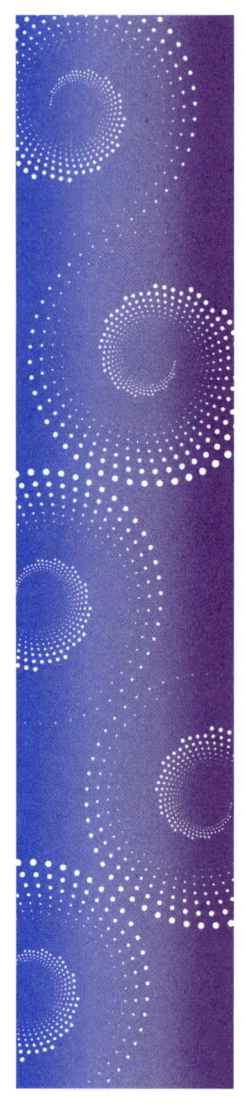

**Life is hard right up until the moment it isn't.**
*Sue Morter*

---○

**Even if you fall on your face, you're still moving forward.**
*Victor Kiam*

> If we had no faults we should not take so much pleasure in noting those of others.
>
> *François de La Rochefoucauld*

> People who say they don't care what people think are usually desperate to have people think they don't care what people think.
>
> *George Carlin*

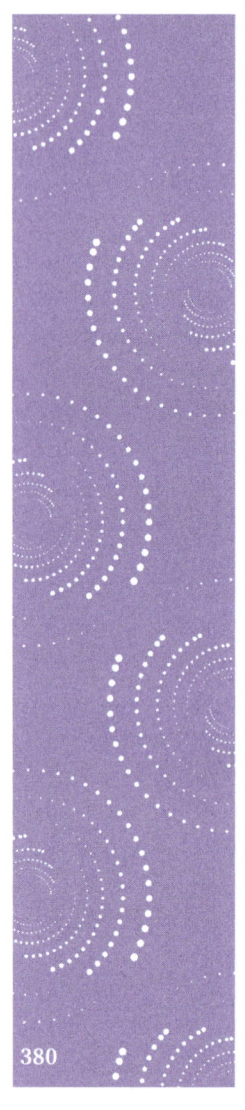

My life is in the hands of any fool who makes me lose my temper. *Joseph Hunter*

---

I may be a living legend, but that sure don't help when I've got to change a flat tire. *Roy Orbison*

The one thing I regret was that my work required an enormous amount of my time, and a lot of travel.
*Neil Armstrong*

To get back to one's youth one has merely to repeat one's follies.
*Oscar Wilde*

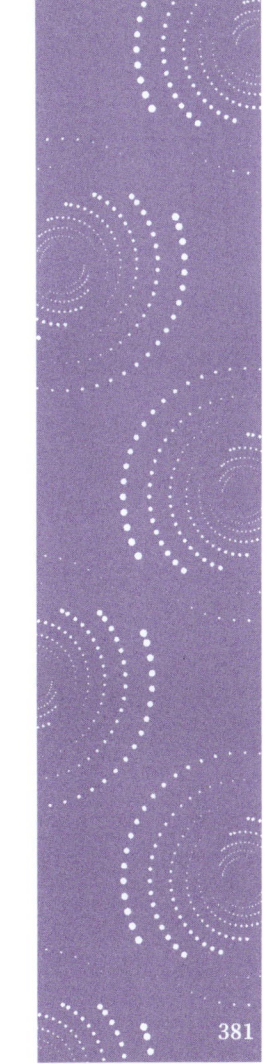

I intend to live forever. So far, so good.
*Steven Wright*

I gave my beauty and my youth to men. I am going to give my wisdom and experience to animals.
*Brigitte Bardot*

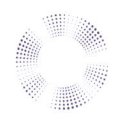
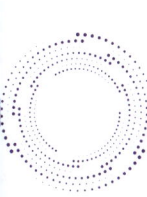

When I hear somebody sigh,
'Life is hard,' I am always
tempted to ask, 'Compared
to what?'
*Sydney J. Harris*

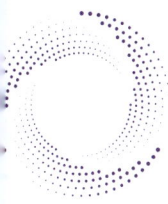

**Why not be oneself?**
**That is the whole secret**
**of a successful appearance.**
**If one is a greyhound, why**
**try to look like a pekinese?**
*Dame Edith Sitwell*

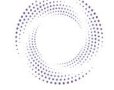

I went to a bookstore
and asked the saleswoman,
'Where's the self-help section?'
She said if she told me, it
would defeat the purpose.
*George Carlin*